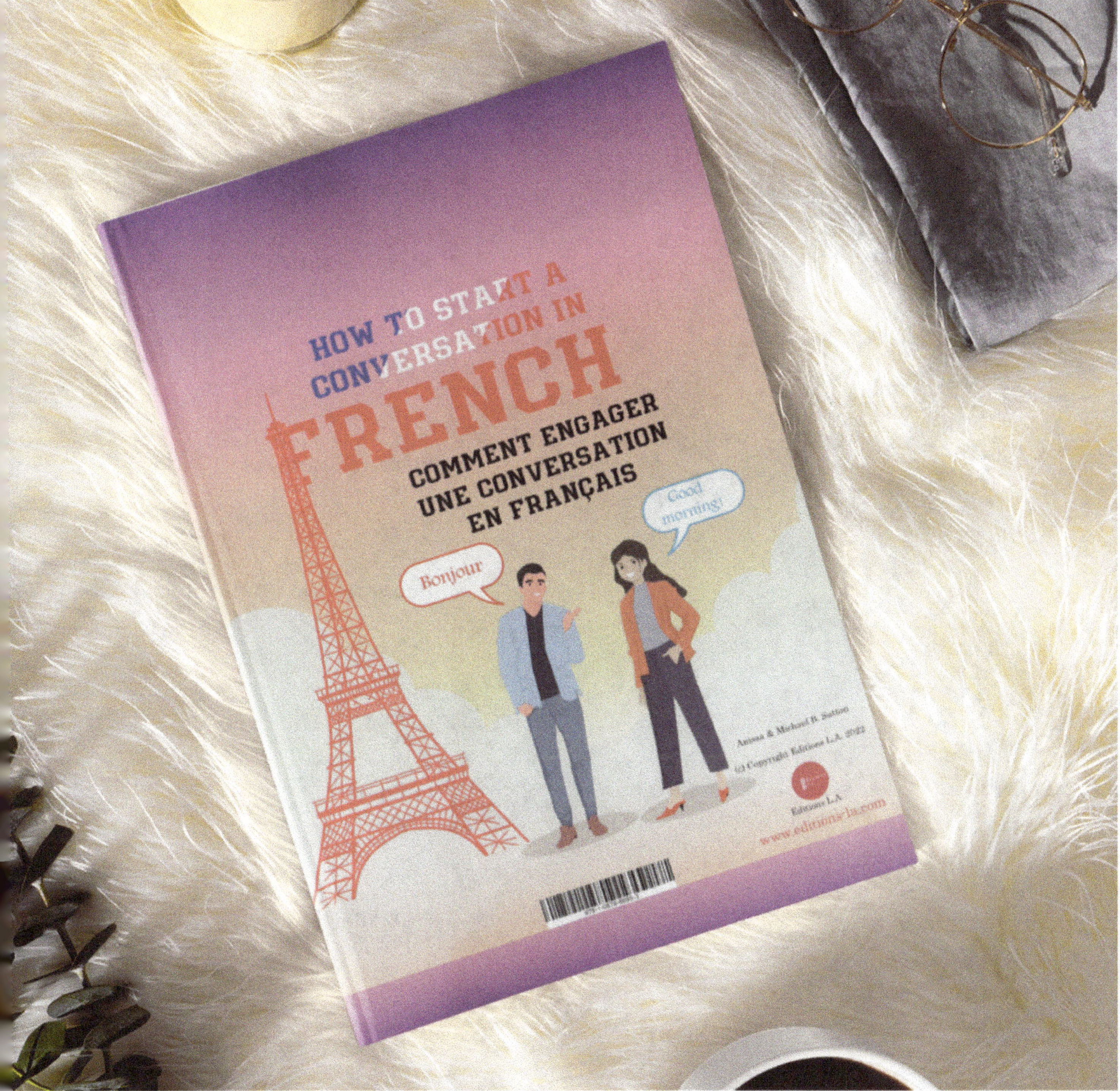

CONTENTS

03 - 34

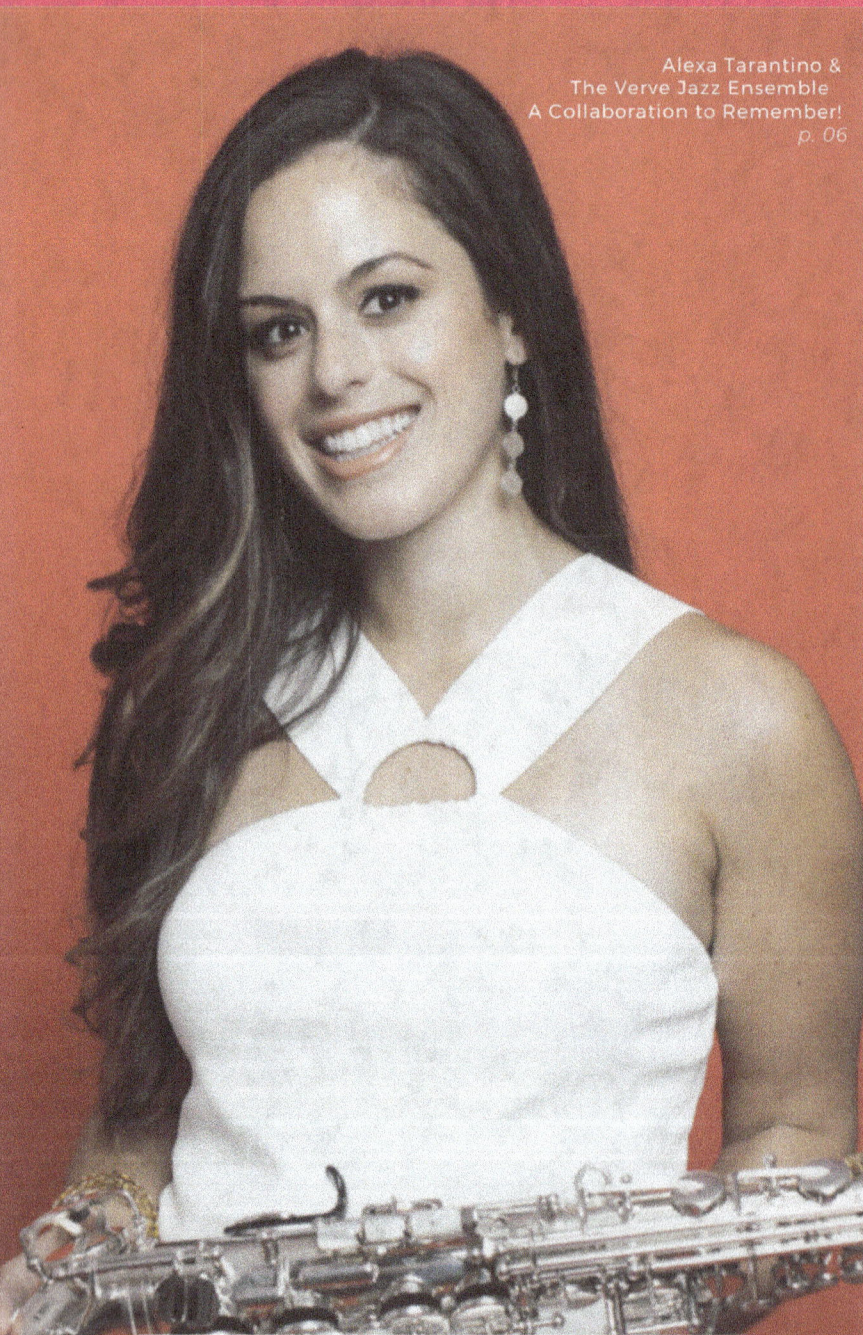

Alexa Tarantino &
The Verve Jazz Ensemble
A Collaboration to Remember!
p. 06

Photos by Anna Yatskevich

06
ALEXA TARANTINO
Celebrating Women's History Month with Jazz Sensation Alexa Tarantino

5
Editor's Note

06-09
Alexa Tarantino
From the Kennedy Center to The Hollywood Bowl, Alexa Tarantino's Journey & The Verve Jazz Ensemble Collaboration

10-21
Women Interviews
Women CEO Insights:
Inspiring Interviews

22 - 25
Doubt No More & How To Say No
5 solutions to elevate your self-confidence
Empowering women in Wellness
Escape the chains: A path to healing and empowerment after narcissistic abuse

25
Fashion
From Basic to Chic
Elevate your style with these simple tips

26-27
Fit & Slim
Set Goals and Crush Them
4 weeks full body workout challenge

28-29
BEAUTY WITHOUT HARM
Try these recipes

30-31
TOP EMPOWERING SONGS
A Must-Add Playlist for International Women's Month

32
TikTok Top Tips
Simple Steps to Grow Your Following

33
MOVIES
Female Filmmakers Making Waves

Pump it up Magazine / 03 - 34

PUMP IT UP MAGAZINE
LINKS

WEBSITE
www.pumpitupmagazine.com

FACEBOOK
www.facebook.com/pumpitupmagazine

TWITTER
www.twitter.com/pumpitupmag

SOUNDCLOUD
www.soundcloud.com/pumpitupmagazine

INSTAGRAM
pumpitupmagazine

PINTEREST
www.pinterest.com/pumpitupmagazine

PUMP IT UP MAGAZINE
30721 Russell Ranch Road
Suite 140
Westlake Village,
California 91362
United States

 (818)514 – 0038(Ext:102)
 info@pumpitupmagazine.com

EDITORIAL

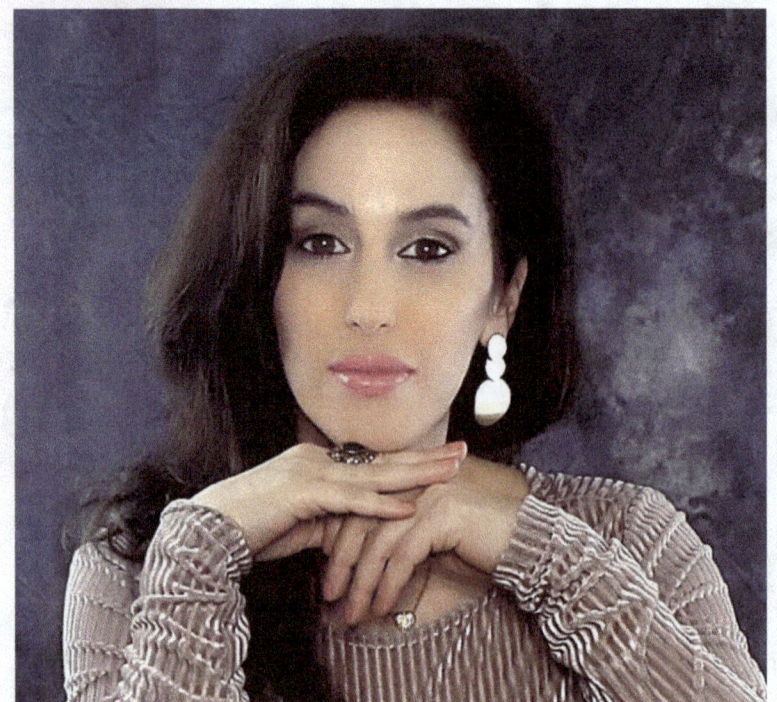

Greetings Readers!

As we celebrate Women's History Month and gear up for International Women's Day on March 8th, the team at Pump it up Magazine is thrilled to present an issue that truly celebrates women in all their glory.

On the cover, we have the immensely talented Alexa Tarantino, whose journey from the Kennedy Center to the Hollywood Bowl is an inspiration to women everywhere who aspire to make their mark in the world of music. Through her collaboration with the Verve Jazz Ensemble, she is breaking down barriers and changing the face of jazz. We couldn't think of a better way to kick off this special issue.

But that's just the beginning. Throughout the pages of this month's issue, we have interviews with inspiring women who are making a difference in their communities and empowering others to do the same.
These women are making waves and changing the world.

We also delve into topics that are important to women's well-being and empowerment. Our wellness section focuses on the importance of creating healthy boundaries in relationships, while our fashion section explores how elevating your style can empower confidence. In our beauty section, we offer tips on enhancing natural beauty with simple recipes.

But we don't stop there. Our fitness section offers advice on creating a plan to achieve your fitness goals, and we shine a spotlight on female filmmakers who are breaking barriers and making their mark in the industry. We also tackle the important issue of C-PTSD caused by narcissistic abuse and offer tools to help women take back their power and overcome this debilitating condition.

We are incredibly proud of this issue and the powerful women who are featured in its pages.

Our hope is that their stories and insights will inspire and empower women around the world to strive for greatness,
and make a difference in their own unique way.

Happy Women's History Month,
and here's to a brighter, more equitable future for all women!

Anissa Sutton

CONTRIBUTORS

FOUNDER
Anissa Sutton

EDITOR
Michael B. Sutton

MARKETING
Grace Rose

PARTNERS

Editions L.A.
editions-la.com

The Sound Of L.A.
thesoundofla.com

Info Music
infomusic.fr

YMC
YourMusicConsultant.Com

BBL
bilingualbookstore.com

WEO
westendorganix.com

Alexa Tarantino

Award-winning jazz saxophonist and woodwind doubler

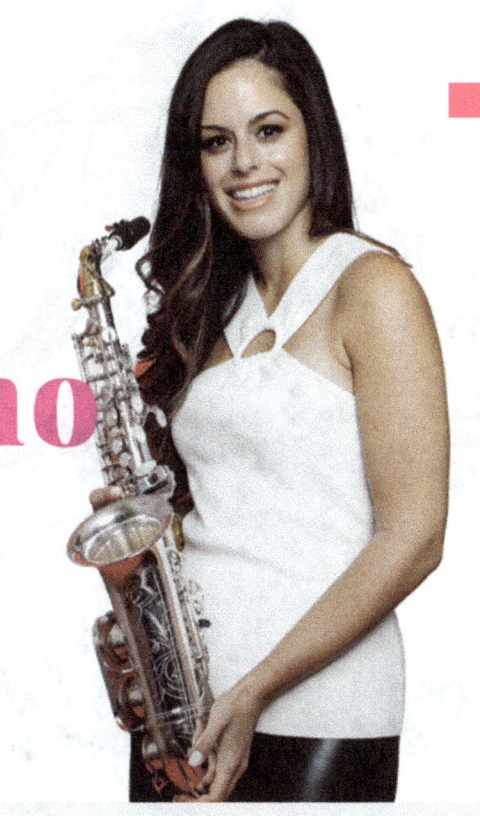

In honor of Women's History Month, we had the pleasure of speaking with Alexa Tarantino, an award-winning jazz saxophonist and woodwind doubler who has established a remarkable reputation in the predominantly male field of jazz.

Having performed and toured with renowned artists such as Wynton Marsalis, Cecile McLorin Salvant, and having a 5-year association with The Verve Jazz Ensemble – including recording on their 2018 number one JazzWeek album, "Connect The Dots" – Alexa has graced some of the world's most prestigious venues and collaborated with a diverse array of top-notch musicians. All of this, while she was completing her Master's Degree in Jazz Studies at The Juilliard School, which she completed in 2019.

Alexa is a rising star in the world of jazz. We spoke to her about her association with the Verve Jazz Ensemble, her experiences as a woman in the industry, her outstanding musical career and achievements, and her aspirations for the future of jazz as an art form.

You made your debut with the Verve Jazz Ensemble on "Connect The Dots" back in 2018. What was your attraction to the group when you were originally approached to join the band by trumpeter Tatum Greenblatt and its leader, drummer Josh Feldstein? Why did you like the VJE's music?

Tatum Greenblatt has been a great friend of mine for years now. We first connected through our work on faculty at Jazz at Lincoln Center's Education Programs. When Tatum comes to me with an idea, I know it's going to be a good one. So when he explained his musical relationship with Josh and VJE, of course I was happy to participate and make music with this new group. Tatum and Josh always choose great repertoire and put together a group of great people.

You've made 3 records with VJE in 5 years, including their latest album "All In" where you played a significant role. The band combines Hard Bop and Latin music, drawing inspiration from composers like Antonio Carlos Jobim. What was your recording experience with VJE like? And how do you feel about the new album and your notable contributions to it?

I love recording in general and am always happy to record for other people's projects because it puts me in a position of learning, growing, and helping someone's vision come to life. Recording for VJE is no different. I appreciate that Josh and Tatum feature me on both alto saxophone and flute, and that they offer me spaces to be featured as a soloist. Every band has its own vibe and trajectory. It's been great to experience their musical choices over the years and to see how the group has developed over time.

ALEXA TARANTINO

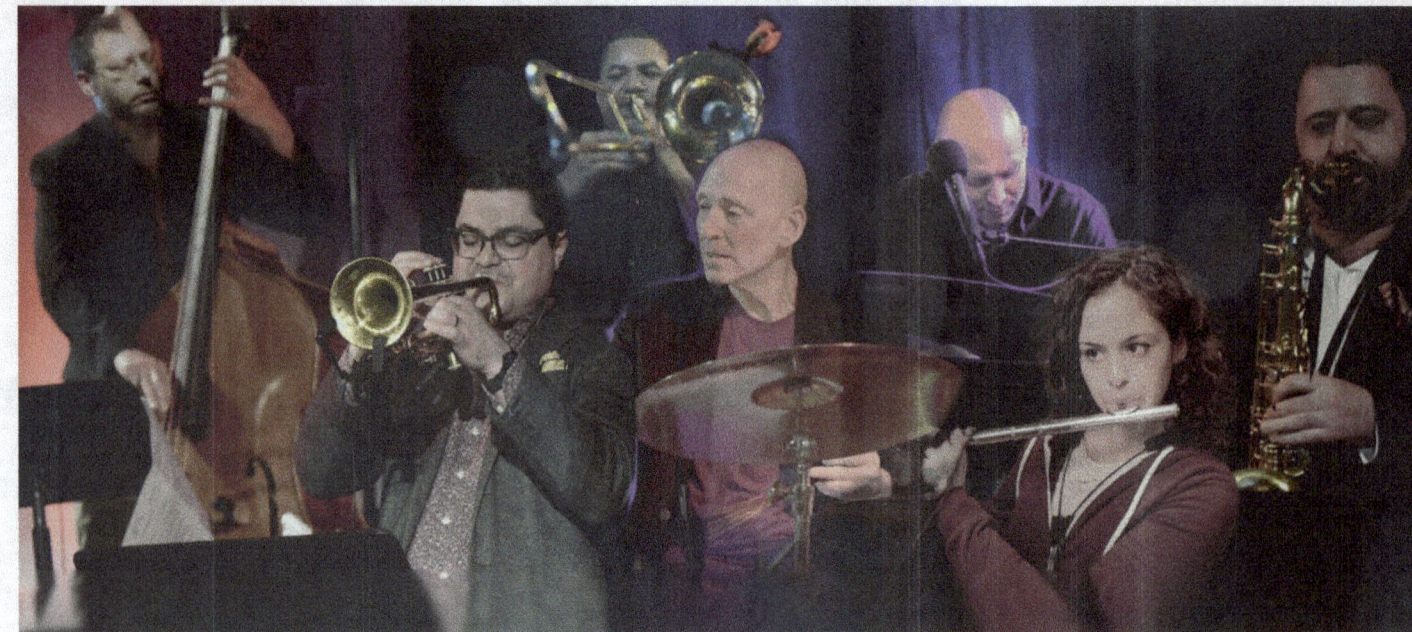

The Verve Jazz Ensemble

As a saxophonist and woodwind doubler, you've worked with diverse ensembles and musicians including the DIVA Jazz Orchestra, Arturo O'Farrill & the Afro-Latin Jazz Orchestra, and your own projects. How have these collaborations helped you express your musical style? What lessons have you gained from working with these talented artists?

It's an honor to collaborate with so many different artists. Each one of them has been an amazing mentor to me. I learn about the history of the music, the importance of staying true to yourself, and the importance of community every time I play.

You've played at prestigious venues like the Kennedy Center and Hollywood Bowl. How do you handle achieving success at a young age while staying grounded in pursuing your artistic goals?

I love to travel and I love to play new venues and new countries. It's something that will never get old. I am consistently humbled by the opportunities that I've had and by the kindness and love that I receive from the people I have met along the way. Plus as a musician you've never "made it", you are always striving to grow and explore something new.

The Verve Jazz Ensemble aims to help the mainstream audience connect with various jazz genres. How has your involvement with The Verve Jazz Ensemble influenced your goal of expanding jazz audience?

The wide range of repertoire and styles recorded by VJE has encouraged me to play whatever music moves me, and to hopefully move others in return. I think when we genuinely play what we love, the audience feels that and appreciates it.

As a female jazz musician in a male-dominated industry, what challenges and opportunities have you faced and how have they shaped your music?

When you are the "only" one in a particular setting, there are often feelings of insecurity, doubt, fear, and comparison that can come along with that. My challenge to anyone experiencing this now is to look at your strengths and what you bring to the table.

How is this community better for having you in it? What do others bring to the table and how can you learn and grow from that?

At the end of the day, my motto has always been to forget about the superficial things, put the time in and do the work, and then just get up on stage and play. Nobody can question that you deserve to be there if you work hard, love to play, are kind, and if you are a positive contributor to that environment.

In Women's History Month, we recognize the impact of female jazz musicians on American history. Who are some that have inspired you, and how have they influenced your music?

Sherrie Maricle, Maria Schneider, Renee Rosnes (and all the women of ARTEMIS), and Terri Lyne Carrington are all present-day role models for me in terms of women in jazz. I also look up to many women who are not necessarily onstage but are behind the scenes producing festivals, venues, and bringing opportunities to artists.
All of these women have inspired me musically and personally. They show us all that there is a place for everyone in this music. It's always inspiring to look back and think about all that women such as Lil Hardin Armstrong, Mary Lou Williams, Melba Liston, and Vi Redd did to move the music further and represent for women in this music.

What does Women's History Month mean to you personally, and how do you hope to use your career to celebrate and uplift women in music and in life more broadly?

Women's History Month inspires me to think about how I can contribute to my community and the world more deeply. I hope to inspire all young students – and specifically young female-identifying students – to follow their dreams, whether that's to play jazz or not. I believe that we all have unlimited potential and I look forward to hearing the next generation of young jazz musicians.

How do you think we can better support young musicians who are interested in pursuing careers in jazz?

Listen listen listen! To as many records and live performances as possible. Soak up everything that your teachers share and never be afraid to ask questions. Your peers will teach you more than you know

For more information about Alexa Tarantino, please visit:

https://alexatarantino.com/

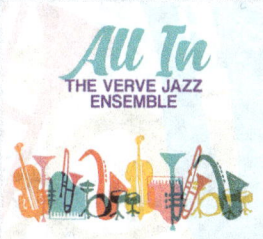

www.verve-jazz.com

The Verve Jazz Ensemble is thrilled to announce the release of their eighth album, "All In," on May 26th.

The album features a collection of two original compositions and eight arrangements of classic and lesser-known material, exploring the theme of "Mid-20th century Americana."

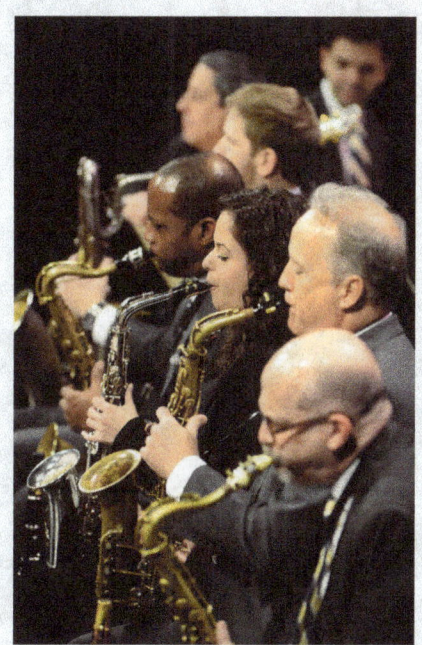

Jazz at Lincoln Center Orchestra Who Is Benny Goodman? Jazz for Young People Concert (Fall 2017)

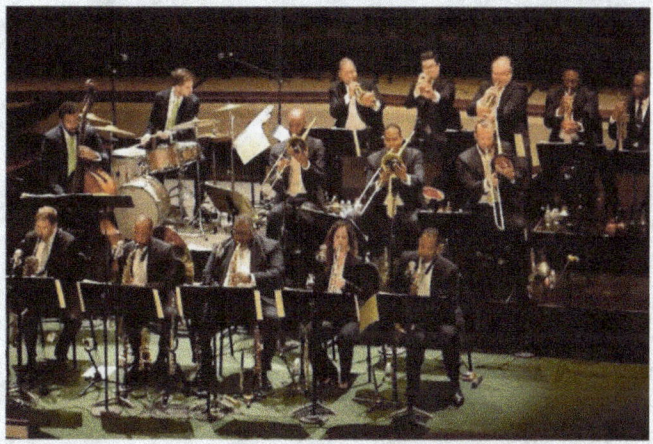

JLCO with Wynton Marsalis at the University of North Carolina Greensboro

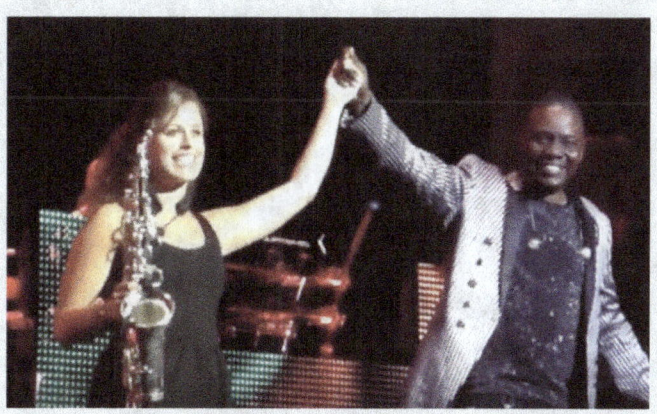

Alexa Tarantino and Philip Bailey of Earth Wind & Fire in Rochester

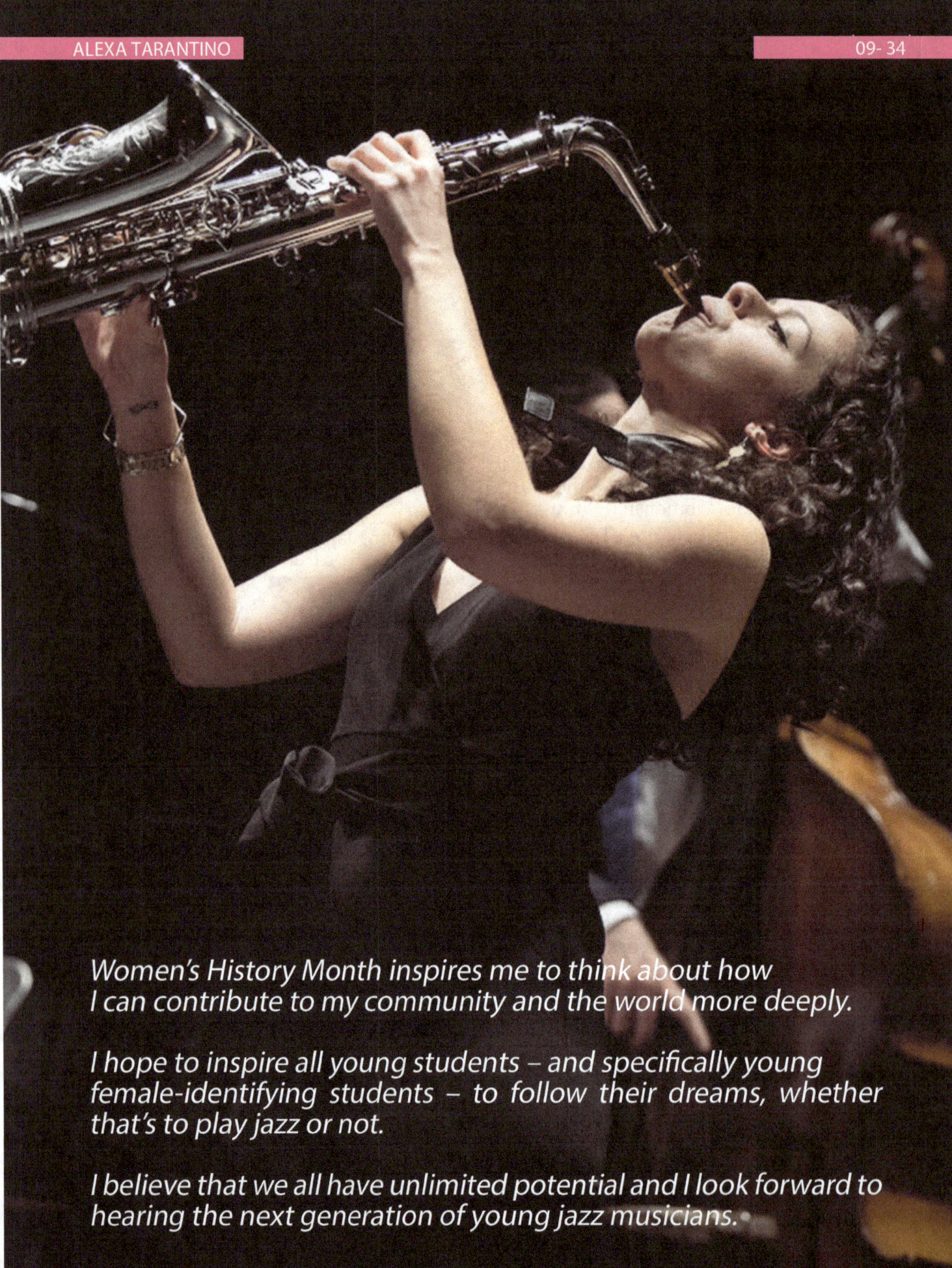

Women's History Month inspires me to think about how I can contribute to my community and the world more deeply.

I hope to inspire all young students – and specifically young female-identifying students – to follow their dreams, whether that's to play jazz or not.

I believe that we all have unlimited potential and I look forward to hearing the next generation of young jazz musicians.

Let's Go Girls!

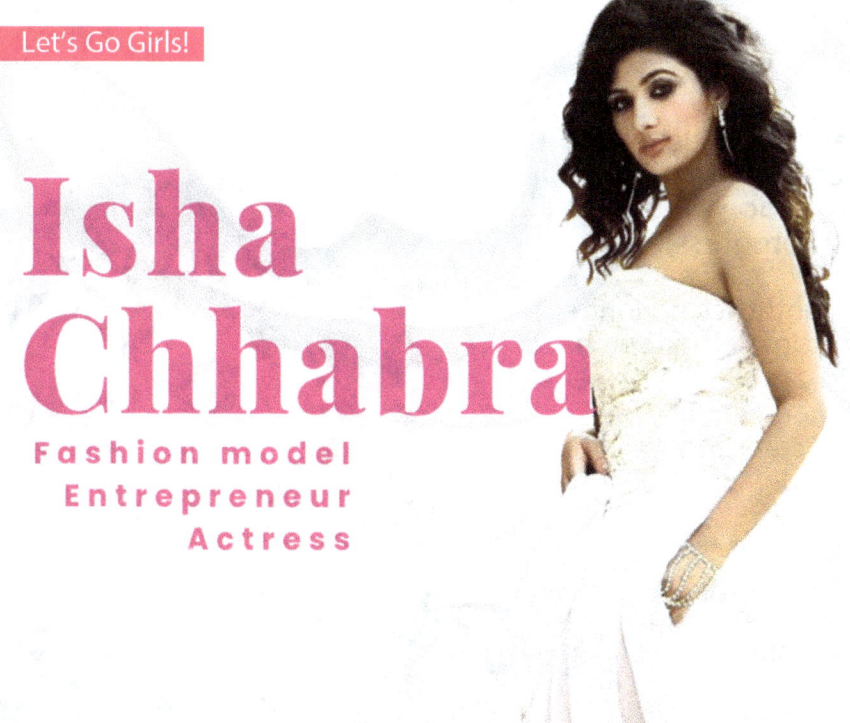

Isha Chhabra
Fashion model
Entrepreneur
Actress

Join us for an inspiring interview with Isha Chhabra - a successful woman who has broken barriers in the entertainment industry through her work in modeling and acting. In this conversation, she shares her journey and what inspired her to pursue a career in the industry. As a woman, she faced obstacles and biases, but she overcame them with perseverance and hard work. She also discusses her entrepreneurial ventures that promote inclusivity and diversity in the industry. As a role model and advocate for women, Isha shares her insights on the progress that the industry has made in terms of promoting equal representation and opportunities for women and what still needs to be done. Finally, she offers valuable advice to aspiring models and actors, shares inspiring moments from her career, and talks about her future goals and plans as a performer and entrepreneur.

Can you tell us about your background and what inspired you to pursue a career in modeling and acting as a woman?

I was into sports, drama, and NCC during my school days. I was performing for a show when I got shortlisted for a TV show on a national channel, and since then, I never turned back. I kept hustling for new adventures and shoots in different cities of my country. My country has cinema in the South, Bengal, and Bollywood. I have worked in South Indian movies before moving to Bollywood, where I appeared on an MTV show, Forbidden Angel, and in a series of MX Player, which got popular during the lockdown and crossed multi-billions views across the world. I moved to Hollywood during the second lockdown of India.

How did being a woman impact your journey in the industry, and what steps did you take to overcome any obstacles or biases you faced?

I love being a woman, and I believe that women have the power to run the world. Women have the brains along with beauty, and beyond that, she is daring to pursue her dream at any cost. I never gave up as a woman because I believe that women are power, a divine source of energy that holds everyone together for the greatest things in life!

As an entrepreneur, can you share with us some of the business ventures you've pursued that promote inclusivity and diversity in the industry?

I have won two of the most prestigious awards of my country, the Maharashtra Gaurav Award by the Road Minister Nitin Gidkari and Gems of North from Punjab Minister Navjot Singh Siddhu. I am also associated with the social campaign, Bird Freedom Day! I would love to spread peace and growth as an entrepreneur. I will connect the whole world under one roof, Ishachhabra network.

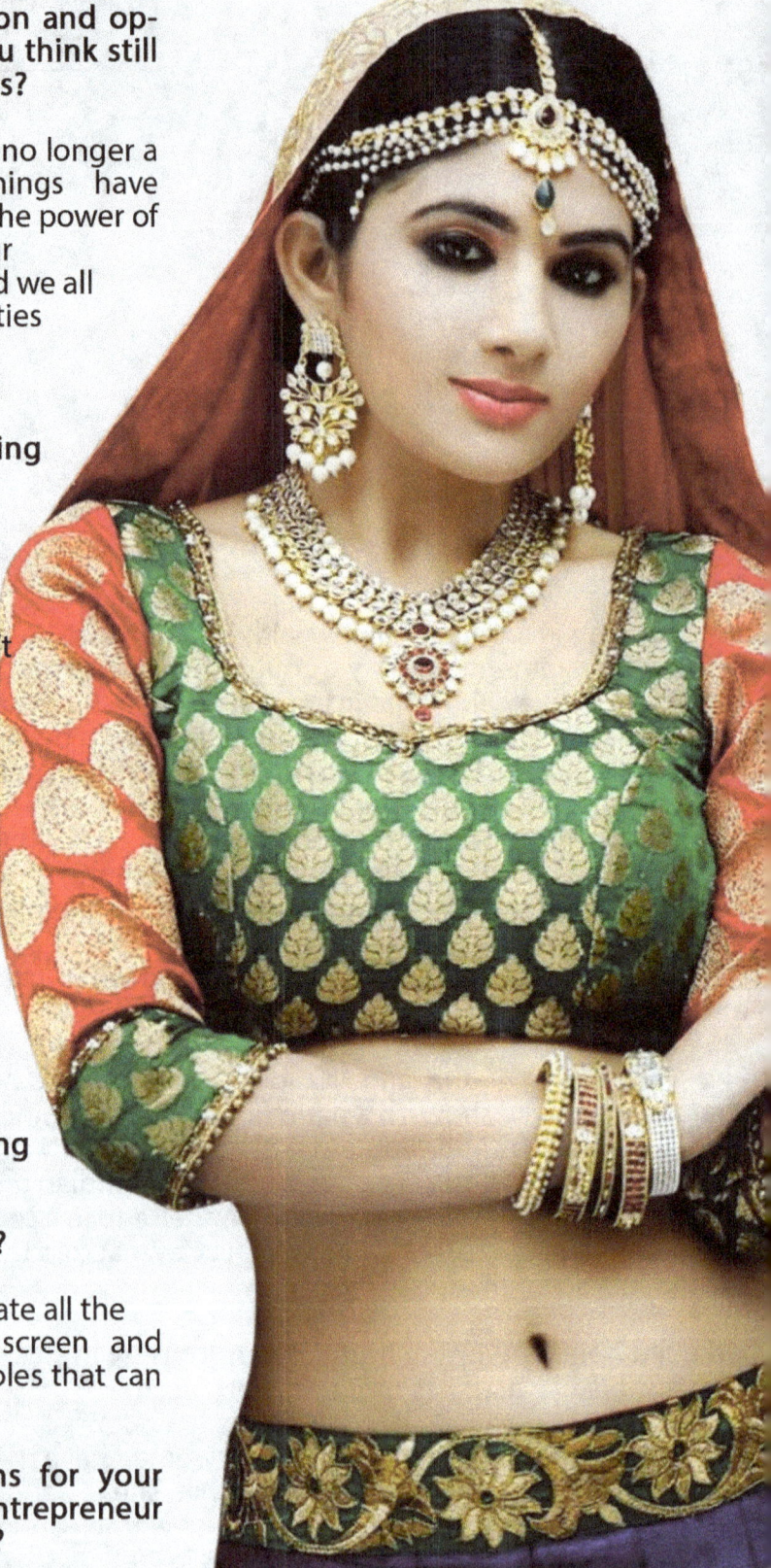

In your opinion, how has the industry evolved in terms of promoting equal representation and opportunities for women, and what do you think still needs to be done to further this progress?

The industry has evolved significantly; it's no longer a man-oriented industry. With time, things have changed for women as the world can see the power of women in every certain way. We handle our responsibilities well with love and care, and we all have equal responsibilities and opportunities these days.

What advice would you give to aspiring female models and actors who are looking to break into the industry and make a name for themselves?

I would just say, please stop paying the wrong people. I request all the freshest females to go through the right path, don't just believe in talk, do research and development (R&D) of the casting people and production. Use all the casting platforms for the casting updates!

Can you share any particularly inspiring or memorable moments from your career as a woman in the indutry?

When I received the Maharashtra Gaurav Award at the India news event, I felt proud of myself!

**How do you use your platform as a successful woman in modeling and acting to ad
vocate for women and promote inclusivity and diversity in the industry?**

Diversity is beauty in our field, and I motivate all the females around me to do better on screen and off-screen. I tend to take more inspiring roles that can offer something to my audience!

What are your future goals and plans for your career, both as a performer and as an entrepreneur who champions women in the industry?

These days, I am just focusing on acting in Hollywood. We are the champions of the industry!

Please visit the following links to connect with Isha Chhabra on social media:
Instagram: https://www.instagram.com/isha_chhabra_slay
Facebook: https://m.facebook.com/IshaChhabraIndia/
Twitter: https://twitter.com/realishachhabra

Glynis Albright
CEO of Glynis' Kitchen

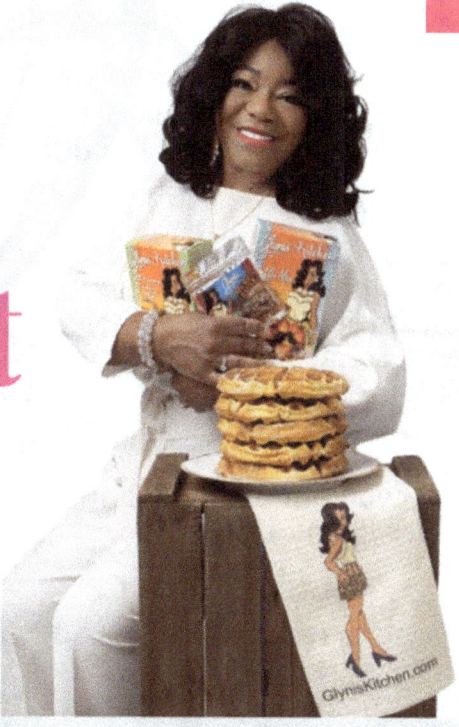

We are thrilled to bring you an inspiring conversation with a remarkable woman today. Glynis Albright, the CEO of Glynis' Kitchen, has turned her passion for cooking and baking into a world-renowned business that motivates women everywhere to chase their dreams and follow their passions.
Despite the challenges she faced, including a rare blood disease, Glynis persevered with her determination and faith to create a thriving gourmet food and wellness brand.
During this interview, she will share her journey, offer guidance to aspiring female entrepreneurs, and emphasize the significance of pursuing your passions and infusing love into everything you do.

Glynis you are an inspiration to many women who dream of turning their passion into a business. Can you tell us about the journey that led you to become the CEO of Glynis' Kitchen?

I was diagnosed with a rare form of leukemia years ago which led me down the nutritional path. My lifestyle and diet had to change which meant not only preparing my meals a certain way but also being careful about my choice of foods. It also meant having a more regimented eating schedule. My relationship with food changed completely. I ate to live, to make my body stronger and to guard it against dis-ease as opposed to eating due to cravings and/or hunger.

You're known as the Waffle Queen, and your food has attracted visitors from all over the word. What motivates you to create such delicious and memorable dishes?

Meeting people who share their health struggles with me really motivate me to create something delicious for them using the nutrients that they need to help with their healing process. It is enough that you are enduring an illness but to be deprived of the things that you love just didn't sit right with me. I felt that it was my Purpose to create foods that would satisfy the palates of those who are "going through a storm" as well. I decided to create gourmet food lines that stayed without certain health guidelines but taste good. I wanted my clients to be healing while eating, instead of making themselves sick because they treated themselves to something that they were once told they couldn't have!

Your success didn't come without challenges. How did you overcome the obstacles that came your way, especially during the toughest bout with leukemia?

One of my biggest hurdles was seeking help from others. I was used to handling things alone, but found myself in a situation where I couldn't control my illness, feelings, or medication effects. I focused on the desire to live and had to accept that I would need assistance with certain tasks. It was tough accepting help from a small group of unexpected, close family members.

Let's Go Girls! 13 - 34

Can you tell us about your natural approach to healing and its connection to Just Sweet Enough® and Cookie Dots®?

My illness led me to carefully consider the food I was consuming. My two gourmet food lines were based on wholesome ingredients like fruits, vegetables, herbs, and spices. I wanted to create treats that had nutritious value and wouldn't cause inflammation for those with health challenges.

How have you balanced your personal and professional life as a wife, mother, and grandmother?

Prioritizing and delegating responsibilities was key. I hired help for my business and a cleaning service for my home. I also learned to say no and prioritize my family first.

What advice do you have for women starting their own business and navigating male-dominated industries?

Just do it! Find your passion, ignore age and gender, and concentrate on yourself. Don't compare, just go for it and give it your all.

How has your PhD in Natural Health/Food Science influenced your business approach?

My education was essential in running my business, as I was able to use math, science, and technology to make Glynis' products a success.

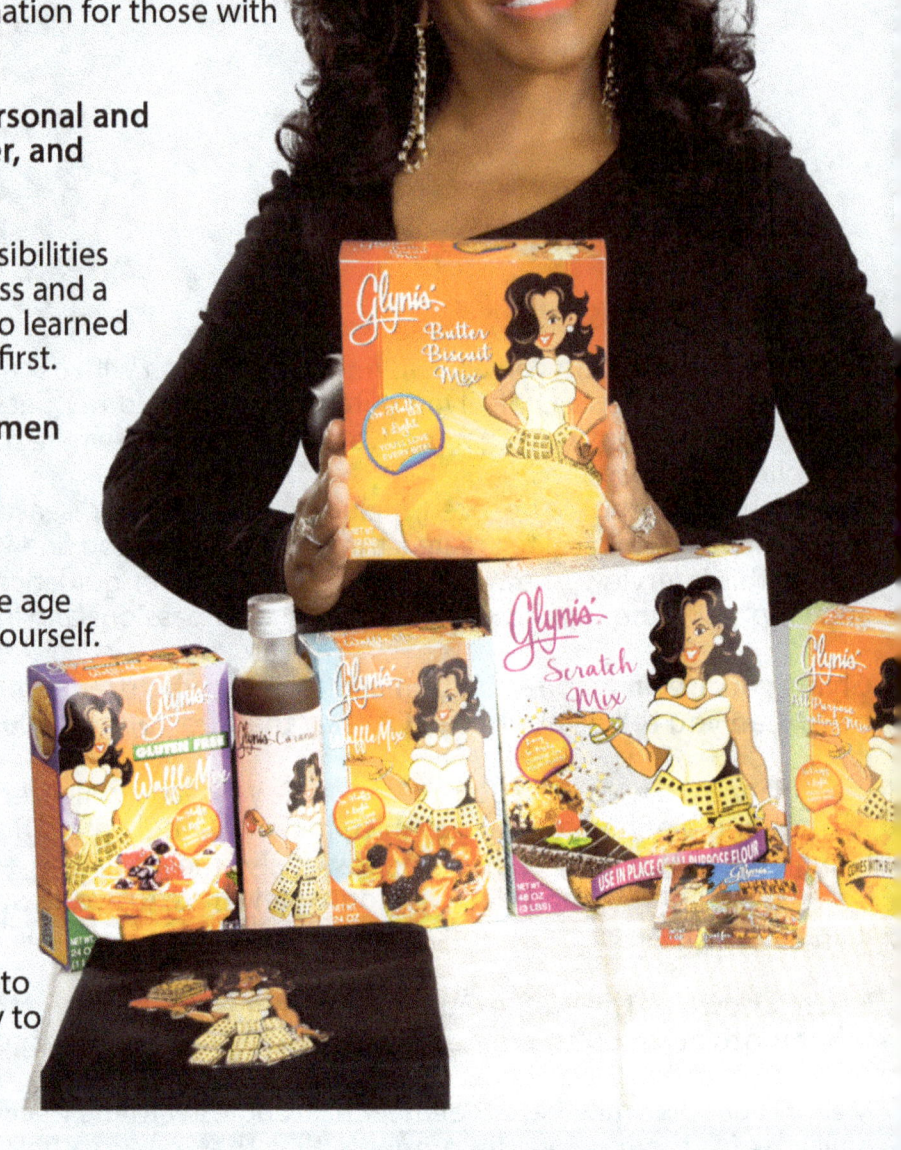

How did you adapt to the challenges of COVID-19 as a small business owner?

Adjusting and prioritizing was crucial. I had to shut down 5 of my food lines and focus on just one - Glynis' Products. Be honest with yourself, do what you can do well, and survive.

Why is it important for women to share their stories of resilience and perseverance?

Sharing stories can help fill someone else's cup and provide encouragement. Share your talents to make a difference and pay it forward.

Visit Glynis website: https://www.glyniskitchen.com
Follow Glynis on social media:
https://www.instagram.com/albrightcuisine
https://www.facebook.com/GlynisKitchenBrand

Paulette Jackson
Author & Entrepreneur

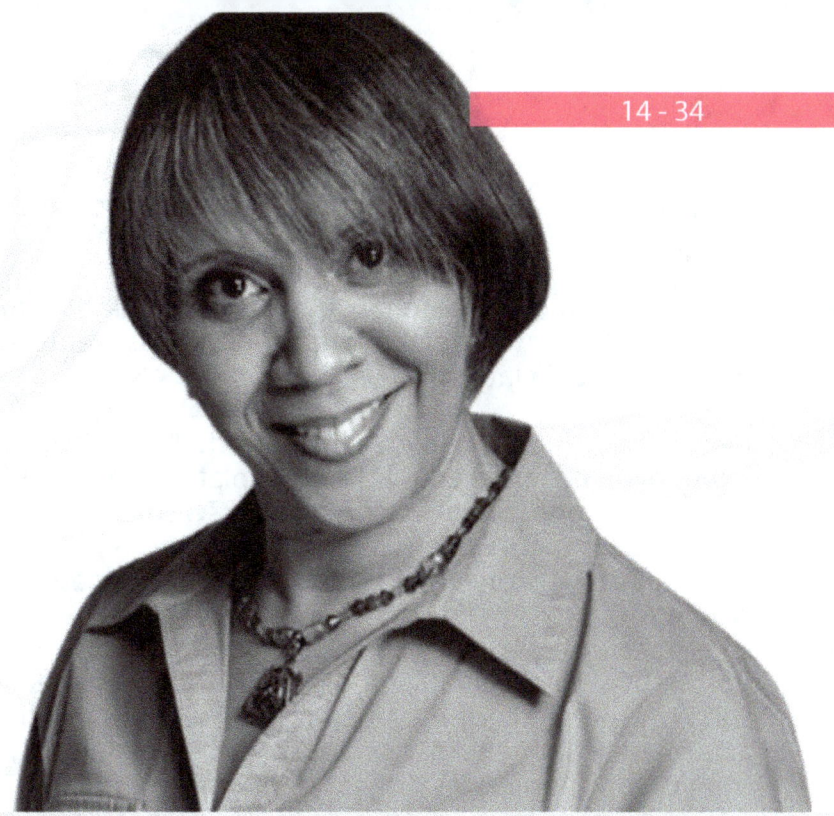

As we celebrate International Women's Day, we had the pleasure of speaking with Paulette Jackson, a successful entrepreneur, author, and radio host. Through her book "My Testimony" and her business ventures, Paulette has overcome adversity and blazed a trail for other women to follow. In this interview, she shares her insights on entrepreneurship, music, and the power of perseverance. Join us as we learn more about Paulette's journey and the lessons she has learned along the way.

Can you share with us more about your personal journey and the challenges you faced as a woman in business?

I've always wanted to be in the arts & entertainment industry, particularly centered around music. In recent years, I got into areas of music and media I never thought I would which lead me to amazing opportunities and connections. Challenges were people not taking me serious as a woman in business, to be heard and prove I was knowledgeable and experienced in this industry.

How did you overcome those challenges and what motivated you to continue pursuing your dreams?

Really what motivated me to pursue my dreams was my love and passion for the arts. I knew working a 9 to 5 for someone else wasn't who I was, sure I did what I had to but in my heart I wanted to be an entrepreneur, to be a creative on my own terms and call my own shots.

Though I do contract work, I still continue to build my brand and take it to new levels.

In your experience, what are some common barriers that women face in business and how can they overcome them?

I don't believe a lot of women have or know about resources that are available that can help them in their business.

Right now, I'm exploring resources I didn't know existed and it's because I started engaging more with other women in business and learning even more than I thought, that I began to start tapping into those valuable resources (grants, certification, etc)

Also, another challenge we as women in business face is being taken seriously by our counterparts but, having the confidence and strength will help overcome those challenges. Knowing our worth is vital.

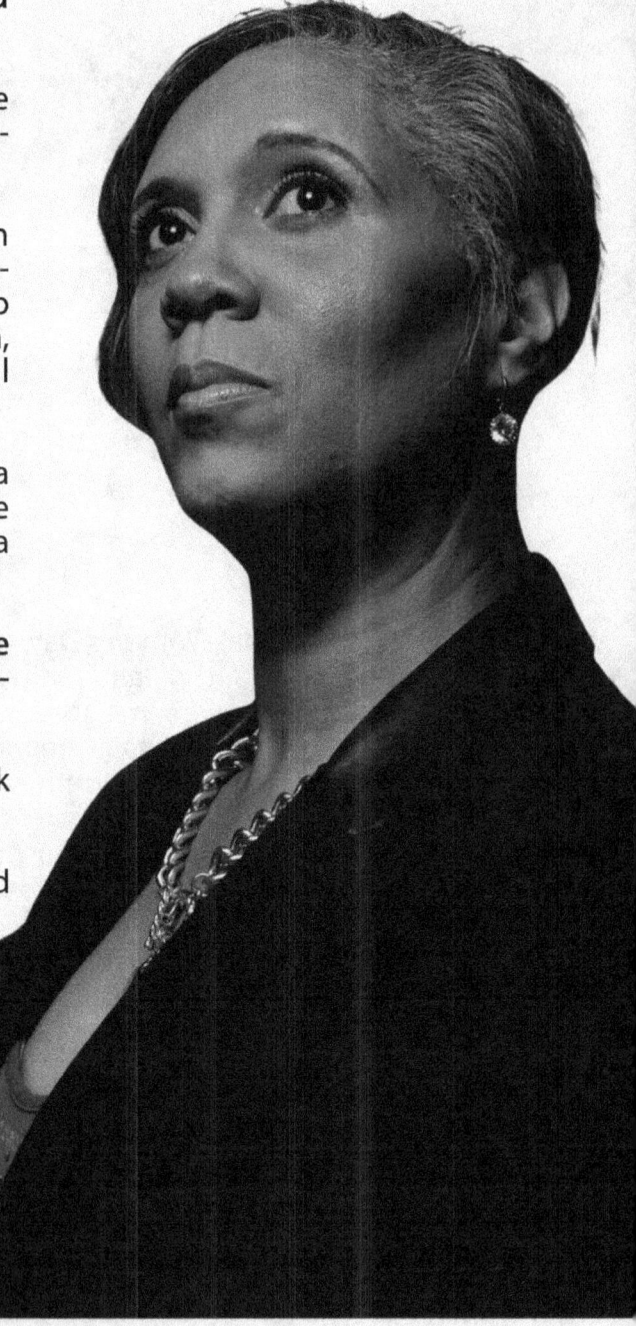

How do you use your platform to advocate for and empower women in the industry?

I use my writing and media platforms to highlight the stories and achievements of women in the arts & entertainment/media industry.

I write for a couple publications, one that focuses on women in Jazz and media, it's a great platform to advocate for women creatives and businesswomen. I also use my own media platforms, including social media, to share the stories and gifts of entrepreneurial women.

I often use my skills as a writer and author to place a spotlight on some of the phenomenal women in the arts & entertainment/media industry who I feel have a tremendous impact. It's my way of honoring them.

How do you prioritize self-care and wellness while running a successful business and managing multiple projects?

Early on, I pushed too hard, so I had to take a step back to rest and recharge.

My business improved because I was more rested and focused. Self-care is important for both personal and business success.

Can you tell us about a project or initiative you are currently working on, and what excites you about it?

I wrote two additional books during the pandemic that I aim to have published and released later this year. I am also looking forward to participating in a panel discussion about self-publication this spring.
I have a few more projects in the works, but I've had to temporarily pause them.
I plan to resume work on them later this year

Can you share any success stories of women you have mentored or worked with who have overcome adversity and achieved their goals?

There's a young lady who has grown her brand so much over the past few years that I've known and worked with. She had some personal challenges which made her have to put her dreams and brand on hold. Even during this challenging time, she still worked on her brand and came back stronger and better than before. She told me a couple times that I was her mentor (I had no idea). Very proud of the progress she has made.

For media inquiries or to learn more about Paulette Jackson and her work, please visit:

Website: www.authorpaulettecjackson.com

Email: inquire@authorpaulettecjackson.com
Phone: (855) 232-9993

Jamie Waryck

CEO
The JW Group
Real Estates Broker

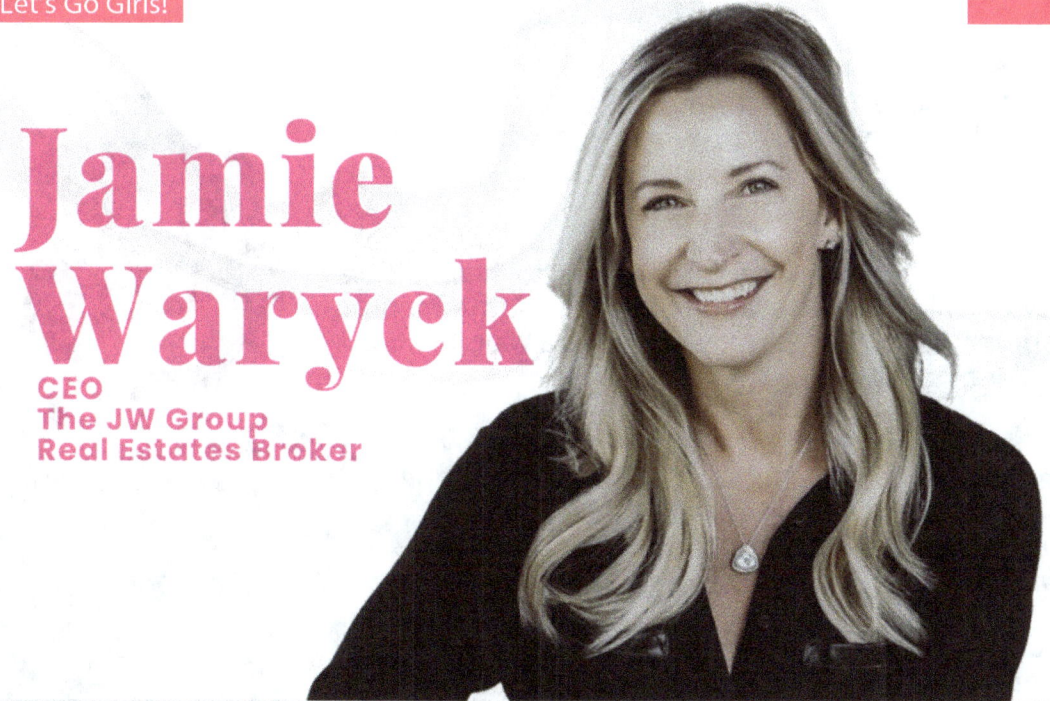

Jamie Waryck, a seasoned real estate broker with over 20 years of experience, has launched her own group, The JW Group, at The Agency. With a focus on providing exceptional real estate services to clients throughout the Southern California region, Jamie and her team are poised to make a significant impact in the industry.

Known for her sharp attention to detail, client-centric approach, and commitment to the highest ethical standards, Jamie has been involved in real estate since 2000, when she launched her career in the Chicago market. Since 2011, she has been working in the Los Angeles area, helping buyers, sellers, and investors navigate the Southern California market, with a special focus on the beach cities of the South Bay.

Jamie's unique background in education and marketing/sales has driven her passion for real estate since she relocated from Chicago to Los Angeles in 2008. She has established herself as a trusted partner throughout the entire real estate process, serving clients in the Greater LA area, including the Beach Cities and Temecula.

"I am thrilled to launch The JW Group and bring my expertise and passion for real estate to clients in Southern California," said Jamie. *"Whether it's a starter condo or a multi-million-dollar estate, I am committed to serving as a trusted advisor and helping my clients achieve their real estate goals."*

With Jamie's wealth of experience, combined with her team's dedication to providing exceptional service, The JW Group is sure to become a leading name in Southern California's real estate industry.

Can you share your journey in the male-dominated field of real estate and what challenges you have faced as a woman in the industry?

There are actually more women than men by numbers in real estate; however, there is no doubt that men do more of the business in most areas. For me, I find there's a good balance between both in the industry and I've always tried to embrace partnerships when they make sense.

As a woman, I have had to think more about my safety in situations than I believe my male counterparts have had to do. I've had to consider the intentions of potential clients through a bit of a different lens. As a woman who doesn't have children, I've probably had more freedom in my schedule than some of my other female counterparts. My schedule has really been my own and that luxury is certainly not lost on me. I have so much admiration for women who hustle in this business and keep their family lives humming along. I truly don't know how they do it.

How have you been able to overcome these challenges and what advice would you give to other women looking to break into the field?

To succeed in real estate, invest in personal development for contract and people skills. Have a clear motivation to help others achieve homeownership. Take education seriously, find a mentor, and build a support system. Success may take over a year in this expensive and challenging industry.

My husband was my support system, and he helped me overcome financial challenges so I could focus on business development. Communication is key to success. *The point is, find your cheerleaders and lean into them along the way. They are your lifeline!*

Can you tell us more about the magazine you owned and operated in Chicago? and how did your experience running a magazine prepare you for a career in real estate?

I launched SIFT Chicago in 2006 to modernize a women's publication for young professionals. However, as digital advertising grew, we struggled to transition from print. Nonetheless, the experience taught me marketing skills and attention to detail that benefit my real estate clients today.

What are the latest trends in LA's real estate market? How do you keep up with them?

Oh goodness, Los Angeles markets are forever and always changing, that is for sure! new laws, rising interest rates, low tory, and influx or exodus of people create constant fluctuations. The only way to stay informed is to be a student of statistics and study the market each day.

How do you see the real estate industry evolving for women in the future and what changes do you hope to see?

I hope to see more women celebrated in real estate for their knowledge, commitment, and skillset. Our world values social media, appearance, and superficial success over hard work and genuine talent. Let's spotlight the real abilities of women in this industr

Can you share any future plans or projects?

Last year, I started The JW Group and plan to build the team further. I'm developing podcast plans, seeking more speaking engagements, and expanding my services for Southern California clients. This dynamic market brings exciting opportunities for us all!

For more information about Jamie and The JW Group:

Please visit her website at: www.JamieWaryck.com
Instagram at https://www.instagram.com/jamiejjw/
Facebook at https://www.facebook.com/Warycksells.

Let's Go Girls! | 18 - 34

Chelsea Davis
Wardrobe Stylist

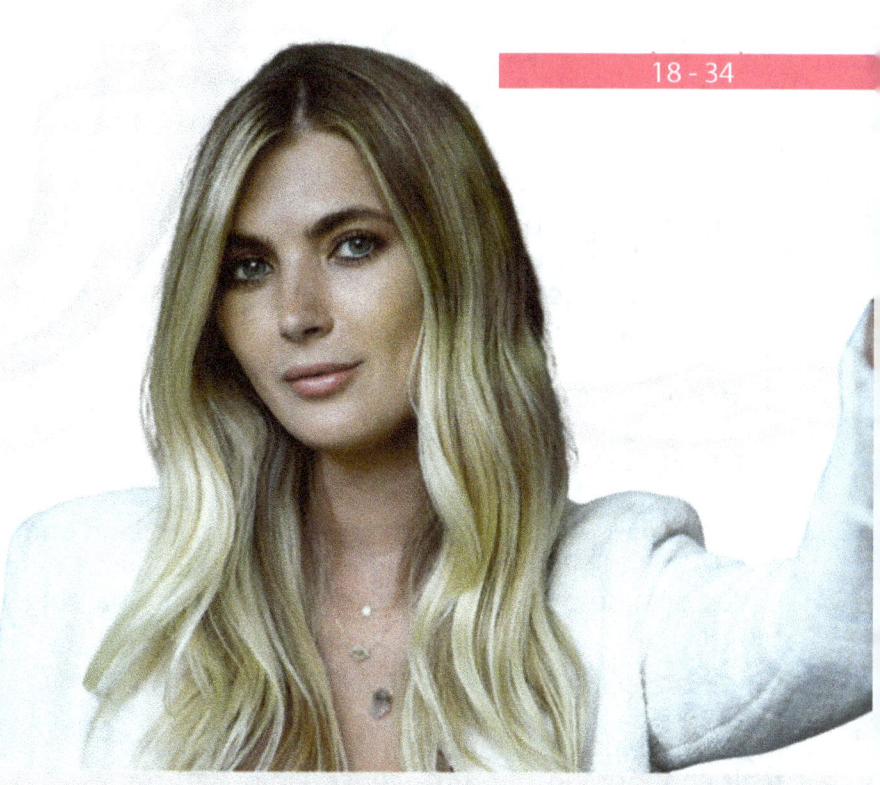

Are you ready to step up your fashion game and create a wardrobe that empowers and inspires you? Look no further, as we sit down with Chelsey Davis, a personal wardrobe stylist who has made a transformative journey from the wholesale fashion industry to a successful travel stylist and closet concierge.

From tips on closet organization to personal shopping and discovering your personal style, this interview with Chelsey will leave you feeling inspired and ready to take on the world with confidence.

Can you share with us your journey to becoming a personal wardrobe stylist and the challenges you faced along the way?

After a decade in the wholesale fashion industry, I transitioned to a personal styling business focused on travel. Despite a major setback with the sudden loss of my mother just two months into my new venture, I took time to care for my family and heal. Through this difficult journey, I have found gratitude and happiness, and am now dedicated to helping others find their personal style and confidence.

How did your background in wholesale fashion shape your approach to wardrobe styling and organization?

Understanding purpose is key in both wholesale and styling worlds. In wholesale, the goal is to assist buyers in selecting the perfect assortment for their customers. In styling, the focus is on the branding story of the boutique or department store and catering to their clientele. My background in wholesale, working with multiple divisions, taught me the importance of organization. The frequent travel required for these brands also allowed me to master packing for any destination and weather.

Can you talk about the concept of being a "Travel Stylist and Closet Concierge" and how you provide unique solutions to your clients?

A "Travel Stylist" styles clients for trips and adventures, ensuring they have a perfectly packed wardrobe ready for any opportunity. Experience freedom and confidence on your next journey with a travel stylist.

As a "Closet Concierge," I fulfill all your closet needs. My passion for solving problems and finding creative solutions makes me an ideal go-to person for clients, whether it's packing for a trip or putting together outfits for the week.

Can you explain your process for creating a "packing package" for clients?

I create packages based on the client's destination and trip length. I offer 4 packages, with the smallest being for a short/long weekend trip and the largest for 14+ days. I offer to compile 3 outfits per day for the chosen package. For example, the smallest package would include 6-9 outfits and the largest 42+ ensembles. I consider the client's activities when compiling outfits.

What sets your services apart from others?

I offer an experience, not just a service. I am a friend and faux therapist to my clients. I share my life experiences and help with any issues outside of style. I bring satisfaction from helping others feel better.

Can you share memorable moments in your career?

My favorite part is witnessing the moment a client feels confident in an outfit I chose. I love getting texts or calls from clients excited about an event or win related to their outfit.

How do you approach closet organization?

I have an intake form that clients fill out before the consultation. During the "Closet Sesh," we discuss goals and try on most of the client's wardrobe to determine what to keep. I guide the client in what is flattering and put together outfits from their existing wardrobe. If needed, a sonal shopping session can be scheduled to add pieces to their closet.

Can you discuss personal shopping in your services?

During the "Closet Sesh," I get to know the client and discuss life goals. I suggest a three-month retainer, but smaller packages are available. Personal style is more than just appearance and can affect the way a person feels. I love personal shopping and helping clients feel confident in their style.

Advice for women pursuing a career change?

Follow what makes you happy. Learn to love yourself and that is the key to a life you love. My two mentors, a life coach and a retired monk, changed my life and showed me how to reprogram my subconscious and live a life of calm, clarity, and compassion.

Future plans and aspirations for your business?

My goal is to continue evoking confidence in women by helping them find their personal style. I hope to add exclusive services such as sound baths and inspire women to love what they do.

Book a consultation with Chelsey at www.CStyle.me to unlock your personal style and travel with confidence.

Let's Go Girls!

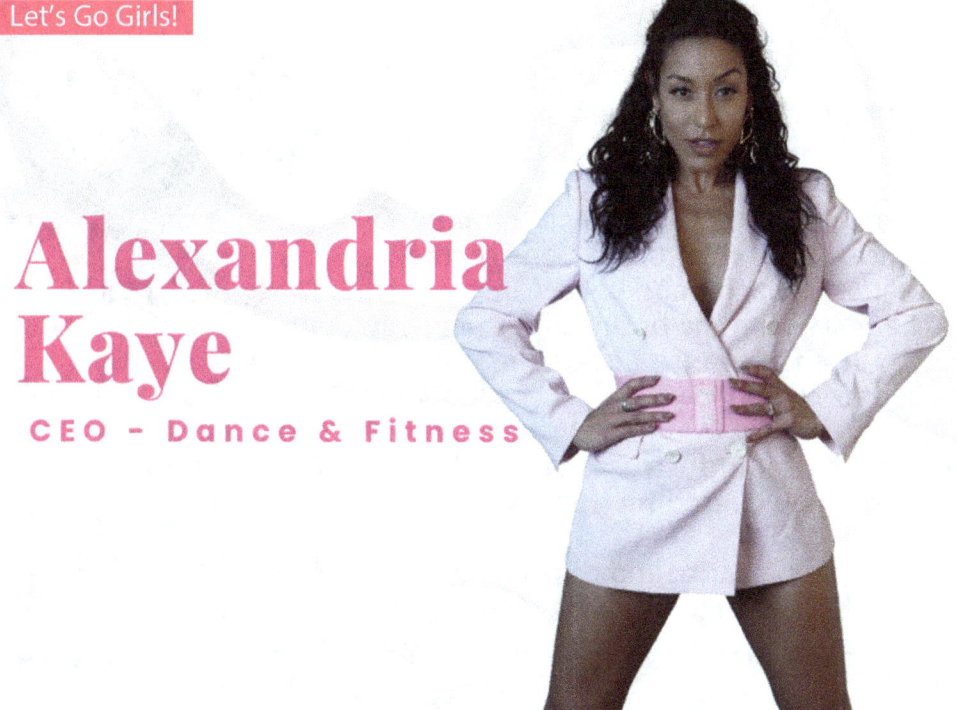

Alexandria Kaye
CEO - Dance & Fitness

FROM PERFORMING WITH LADY GAGA, J-LO, USHER, CHRIS BROWN AND LANA DEL REY TO LEADING TEAM3XT AS CEO: ALEXANDRIA KAYE'S JOURNEY AS A TRAILBLAZER IN DANCE AND EMPOWERMENT

Alexandria Kaye, Chief Performance Officer for Team3XT, has been inspiring and empowering women through dance and fitness for years. With her background in yoga and fitness, her approach to dance and performance is rooted in being present and mindful, incorporating breath-work and meditation into her work with Team3XT. Kaye's commitment to creating a safe and supportive environment for women has made her a leader in the dance industry.

Kaye's career in dance has taken her to some of the biggest stages in the world, including her performance with Lady Gaga at the Super Bowl halftime show, which was a dream come true. Working with other high-profile artists such as Lana Del Rey has been a source of inspiration and creativity for Kaye, elevating her visions and ideas to new levels of meaning.

As a woman in a male-dominated industry, Kaye has faced her fair share of challenges, but her dedication to her craft and her determination to succeed have been unwavering. She has overcome these obstacles by continuing to train and work on her skills, and by surrounding herself with a supportive community of women.

Kaye's mission with Team3XT is to promote women's empowerment through dance and fitness, creating a community where women can thrive and break past their limitations. The transformation she sees in the women who complete even just one quarter of the Team3XT Performing Company is truly inspiring, as they gain confidence, community, and the courage to speak up in their personal and professional lives.

Balancing the demands of working with high-profile clients while managing her role as Chief Performance Officer for Team3XT can be challenging, but Kaye has learned to prioritize, stay organized, and be adaptable. She has also learned the importance of being prepared, positive, and fun to work with, which has served her well in her collaborations with high-profile artists.

In conclusion, Alexandria Kaye is a true trailblazer in the dance industry, using her passion and expertise to empower and inspire women everywhere. With her work at Team3XT, she is changing lives and promoting women's empowerment through dance and fitness, making a positive impact in her local community and on a broader scale.
day.
Nothing inspires me like being told I can't do something!

Let's Go Girls!

What inspired you to pursue dance and become C.E.O for Team3xt?

Growing up, I was surrounded by music and dance through my family, inspiring me to pursue a career in entertainment. I'm drawn to the challenge and dedication of dance, and believe in its physical, mental, and spiritual benefits. With my business partner Ferly Prado, we founded Team3xt to make dance accessible to all, regardless of age, body type, or background.

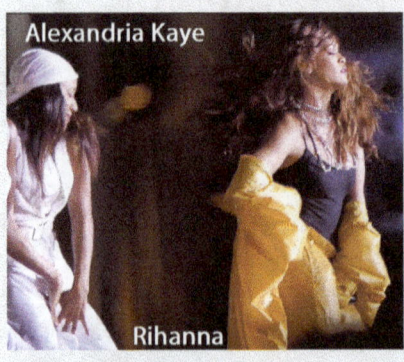

As a woman in a male-dominated industry, what challenges have you faced and how have you overcome them?

Challenges like maintaining my appearance and risk of being fired due to personal reasons have been overcome by training and improving my craft. I stay professional, even during difficult situations.

How do you inspire and empower the women you work with at Team3xt and in your professional network?

I empower women with fearlessness and positivity, living by the quote, "Be fearless in the pursuit of what sets your soul on fire." Self-care is important, and I encourage it. Our supportive community at Team3xt is a major factor in our success.

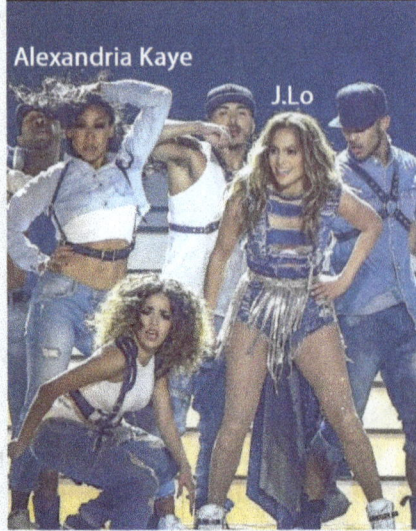

What was it like performing with Lady Gaga for the Super Bowl halftime show, and how did that experience impact your approach to dance and performance?

Performing with Lady Gaga for the Super Bowl was a dream come true and one of the highlights of my career. It was an incredible experience to perform on such a big stage, with over 100 million viewers and surrounded by my closest friends and colleagues.

The energy of the audience was electric, and it taught me the importance of always being prepared and staying in the moment during a performance. This experience reinforced my belief in the value of hard work and dedication, and I strive to instill these values in my students.

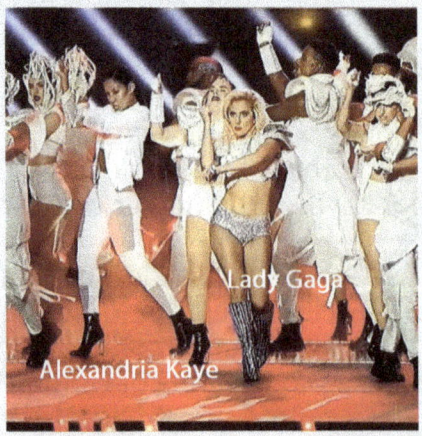

You've had the opportunity to work with many talented artists throughout your career, including Lana Del Rey. What do you find most inspiring about collaborating with other creatives, and how does that impact your work with Team3xt?

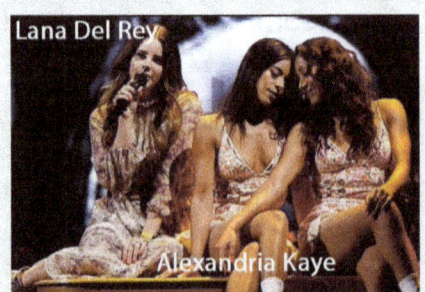

Collaborating with other creatives is always a unique and inspiring experience. Working with others elevates your own ideas and helps bring new perspectives to your work. I find that working with a team or partner produces better outcomes, and I believe that this is true not only in the dance industry, but in all areas of life. My experiences working with talented artists have reinforced the importance of teamwork and collaboration, and I strive to instill these values in the women I work with at Team3xt.

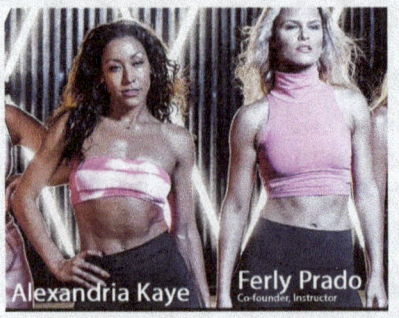

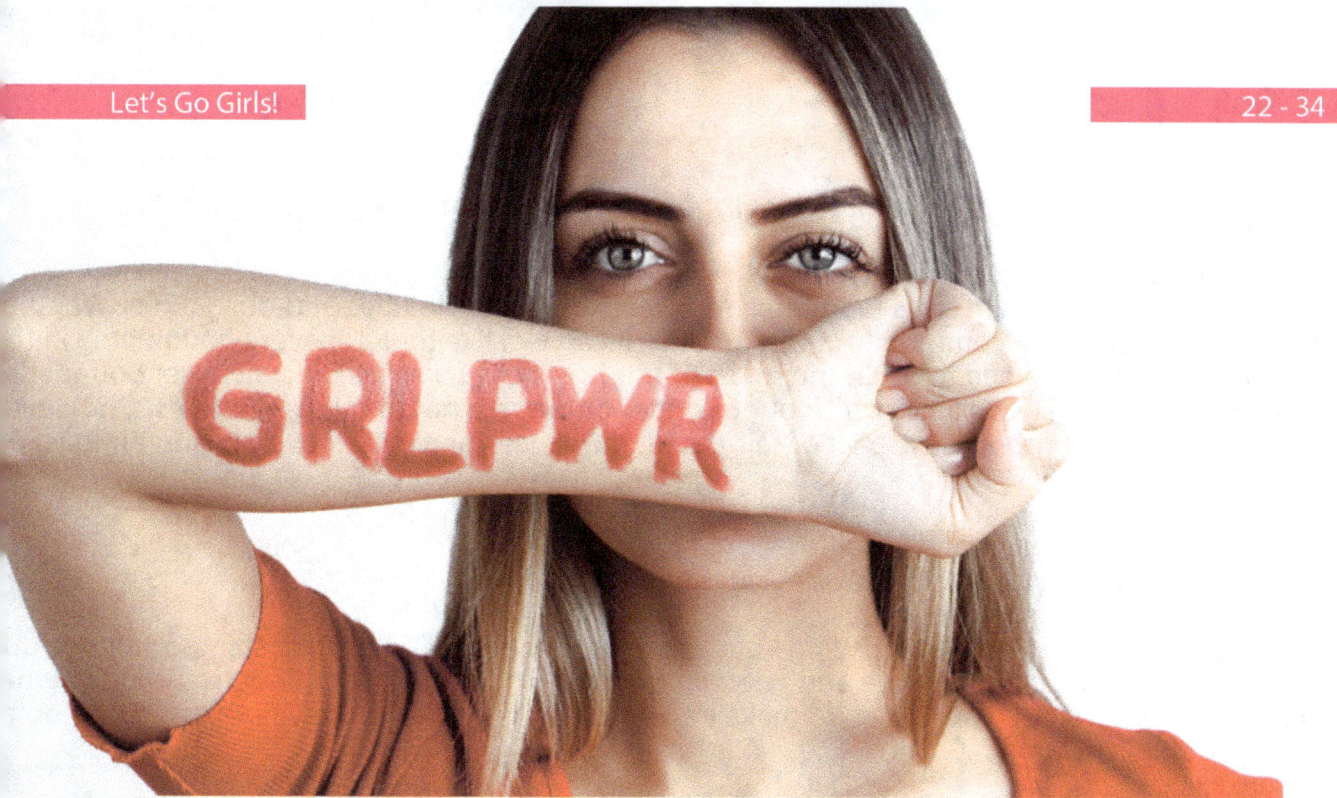

DOUBT NO MORE:
5 SOLUTIONS TO ELEVATE YOUR SELF-CONFIDENCE

Self-confidence is a crucial aspect of our lives that affects how we interact with others, perform tasks, and approach challenges. However, many people struggle with feelings of insecurity, self-doubt, and low self-esteem. These negative emotions can prevent us from reaching our full potential and hinder our personal and professional growth.

If you're one of the many people who struggle with self-confidence, don't worry. There are several practical solutions that can help you elevate your self-esteem and increase your confidence levels. Here are five of the most effective ways to do so:

Practice Self-Care: Taking care of your physical and mental well-being is essential for boosting your self-confidence. Engage in activities that make you feel good, such as exercise, meditation, or reading a book. Additionally, make sure to get enough sleep, eat a healthy diet, and avoid negative self-talk.

Set Realistic Goals: Setting achievable goals for yourself can help you feel more confident and in control. Start small and gradually increase the difficulty of your goals as you progress. Celebrate your successes along the way, and don't beat yourself up over failures.

Surround Yourself With Positive People: Surrounding yourself with supportive, positive people can help boost your self-confidence. Seek out friends, family members, or co-workers who are encouraging and uplifting, and limit your time with those who bring you down.

Learn New Skills: Learning new skills can help you feel more confident and competent. Take up a new hobby, enroll in a course, or attend workshops. The sense of accomplishment that comes with mastering a new skill can help boost your self-esteem and confidence.

Accept Your Flaws: Nobody is perfect, and accepting your flaws is a crucial step in building self-confidence. Instead of trying to hide or change your imperfections, embrace them and focus on your strengths. Remember that your flaws are what make you unique and special.

In conclusion, self-confidence is a vital aspect of our lives that affects our personal and professional growth. By practicing self-care, setting realistic goals, surrounding yourself with positive people, learning new skills, and accepting your flaws, you can elevate your self-esteem and increase your confidence levels. Don't let self-doubt hold you back. Start taking steps today to become the confident, self-assured person you've always wanted to be.

HOW TO SAY NO!
The Art of Saying No: Empowering Women in Wellness

I. "The Importance of Saying No in Wellness"

As women, we often find ourselves juggling a multitude of responsibilities and obligations. Whether it's work, family, friends, or community commitments, it can feel like there's never enough time in the day to do everything we need to do. In the midst of this busyness, it can be difficult to set boundaries and say no to things that don't align with our priorities or that are not in our best interests. However, learning to say no is an important aspect of self-care and wellness, and it can have a positive impact on our overall well-being.

II. Understanding Your Values and Priorities
"Putting Yourself First: Understanding Your Values and Priorities"

The first step in saying no is understanding your values and priorities. What is most important to you? What do you want to focus your time and energy on? When you have a clear understanding of what matters most to you, it becomes easier to make decisions that align with your values and to say no to things that don't.

III. The Strength of Saying No
"Saying No is a Sign of Strength: Embracing Your Power"

Next, it's important to recognize that saying no is not a sign of weakness or selfishness. In fact, it's a sign of strength and self-awareness. When we say no, we are taking control of our time and our lives, and we are putting ourselves and our well-being first. This can be especially difficult for women, who may feel pressure to put others first and to take on more than they can handle. However, it's important to remember that taking care of ourselves is not only necessary for our own well-being, but it also allows us to be more present and effective in our other relationships and responsibilities.

IV. Practicing Assertiveness
"The Power of Assertiveness: Expressing Your Needs and Boundaries"

When it comes to actually saying no, it can be helpful to practice assertiveness. This means expressing your needs and boundaries in a clear and confident manner. You can start by using "I" statements, such as "I can't commit to that right now" or "I need to prioritize my time differently." It's also important to be firm and not give in to guilt or pressure from others.

V. Strategies for Managing Time and Setting Boundaries
"Setting Boundaries: Strategies for Managing Your Time"

In addition to assertiveness, it can be helpful to have some strategies in place for managing your time and setting boundaries. This might include setting aside time for self-care, such as exercise, meditation, or simply relaxing, and saying no to commitments that interfere with this time. It can also mean delegating tasks, outsourcing where possible, and learning to prioritize your to-do list.

VI. Embracing the Process
"The Art of Saying No: A Journey of Self-Discovery"

Finally, it's important to remember that saying no is a process, and it can take time to get comfortable with it. Be patient with yourself, and remember that it's okay to make mistakes. The most important thing is to keep practicing and to continue putting yourself and your well-being first.

VII. Conclusion
"Taking Control of Your Life: The Benefits of Saying No"

In conclusion, saying no is an important aspect of self-care and wellness for women. By taking control of our time, our lives, and by setting boundaries, we can create more space for the things that matter most to us, and we can live with purpose, intention, and joy!

ESCAPE THE CHAINS!

A Path to Healing and Empowerment after Narcissistic Abuse

Narcissistic abuse is a serious issue that affects millions of people around the world. It is a form of psychological abuse that can have devastating effects on a person's mental and emotional well-being. People who have been subjected to narcissistic abuse often feel trapped, helpless, and alone. However, there is hope for those who are ready to break free and reclaim their power. In this article, we'll explore the path to healing and empowerment after narcissistic abuse.

Understand the Dynamics of Narcissistic Abuse

The first step in escaping the chains of narcissistic abuse is to understand what it is and how it works. Narcissistic abuse is a pattern of behavior used by a narcissistic individual to manipulate and control their partner. This behavior often involves verbal and emotional abuse, gaslighting, and other forms of manipulation. The goal of the narcissistic abuser is to make their partner feel small, inadequate, and dependent on them. This creates a dynamic in which the victim becomes trapped and feels unable to leave the relationship.

Seek Professional Help

If you're ready to escape the chains of narcissistic abuse, it's important to seek professional help. A therapist or counselor can help you understand the dynamics of the relationship and provide support as you navigate the healing process. They can also help you develop coping skills and strategies for dealing with the aftermath of the abuse.

Join a Support Group

Another important step in escaping the chains of narcissistic abuse is to join a support group. Support groups provide a safe and supportive environment where you can connect with others who have experienced similar situations. You can share your experiences and learn from others who have been through similar challenges. Support groups can also provide a sense of community and help you feel less alone as you navigate the healing process.

Practice Self-Care

Self-care is essential for healing after narcissistic abuse. This means taking time for yourself, engaging in activities that bring you joy, and focusing on your physical, emotional, and mental health. Self-care can include activities such as exercise, meditation, journaling, or simply taking a relaxing bath. It's important to prioritize self-care and make it a regular part of your routine.

Create Boundaries

Creating boundaries is an important step in empowering yourself after narcissistic abuse. This means setting limits on what you will and won't tolerate from others, including the narcissistic individual. It's important to communicate these boundaries clearly and stick to them, even if it means saying no or walking away from the relationship.

Conclusion

Escaping the chains of narcissistic abuse is a journey of healing and empowerment. It takes time, effort, and support, but it is possible. By understanding the dynamics of narcissistic abuse, seeking professional help, joining a support group, practicing self-care, and creating boundaries, you can reclaim your power and take back control of your life. Remember that healing is a process, and it's okay to take things one step at a time.

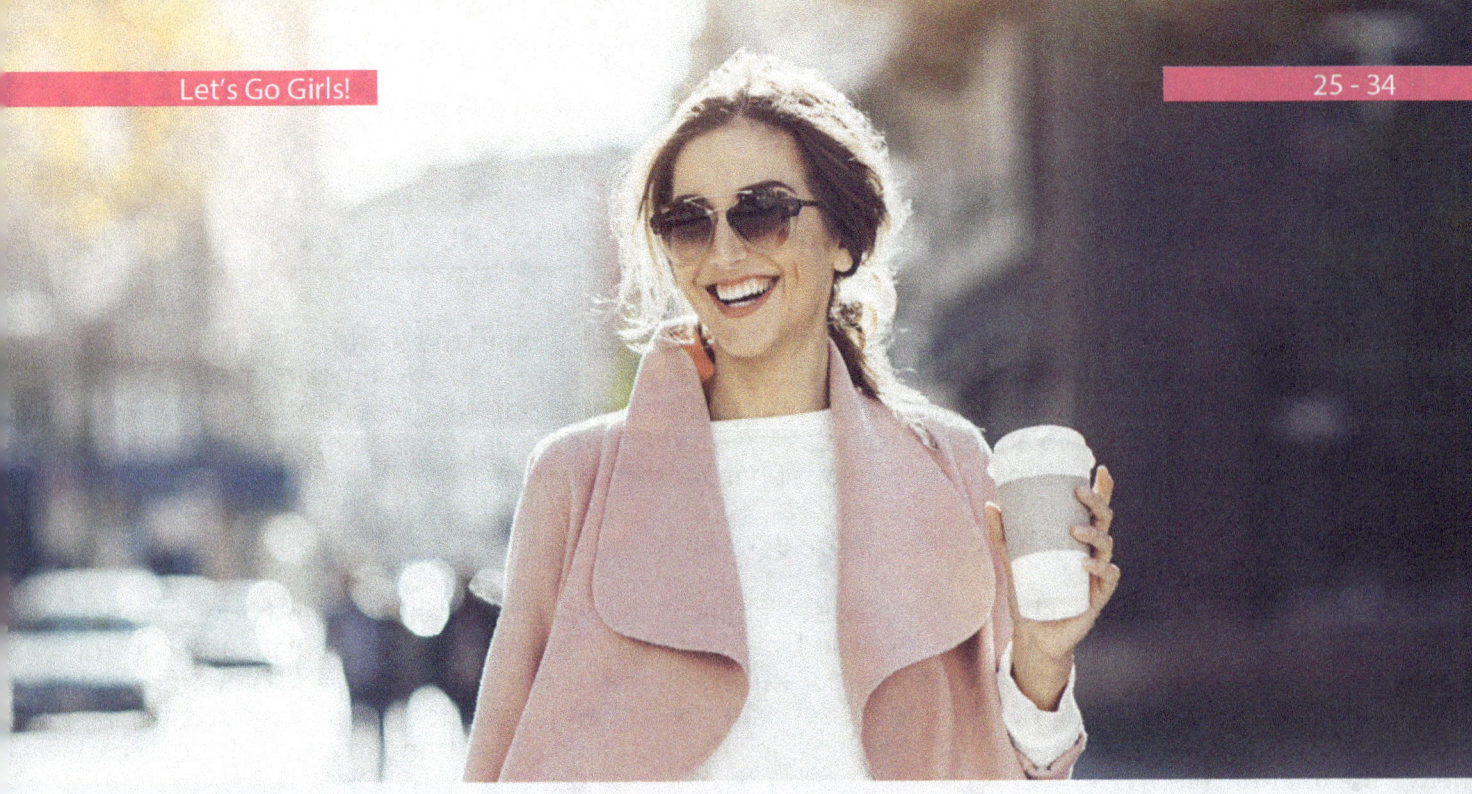

FROM BASIC TO CHIC: ELEVATE YOUR STYLE WITH THESE SIMPLE TIPS

Are you tired of feeling like your style is stuck in a rut? If you're looking to upgrade your wardrobe and take your look from basic to chic, you've come to the right place. In this article, we'll provide tips and tricks to help you elevate your style and look your best, no matter the occasion.

Invest in Quality Pieces
One of the keys to elevating your style is investing in quality pieces that will last. Look for pieces made from high-quality materials that are well-constructed and will hold up over time. These pieces will not only look better, but they will also last longer, saving you money in the long run.

Experiment with Trends
While it's important to invest in quality pieces, it's also important to have fun and experiment with new trends. Look for pieces that will complement your personal style and that you feel comfortable wearing. If you're not sure where to start, try incorporating a trendy accessory, like a statement necklace or a bold scarf, into your look.

Accessorize
Accessories can make all the difference when it comes to elevating your style. Consider adding a statement piece, like a statement necklace or a bold scarf, to your look to add some extra flair. You can also invest in a high-quality handbag or pair of shoes to complete your outfit.

Pay Attention to Fit
The fit of your clothes is just as important as the pieces themselves. Make sure your clothes fit properly and are not too tight or too loose. This will not only make you look more put-together, but it will also help you feel more confident and comfortable.

Experiment with Layering
Layering is a great way to add depth and interest to your look. Try layering different pieces, like a blazer over a t-shirt or a sweater over a collared shirt, to create a chic and sophisticated look.

Invest in Tailoring
If you're struggling to find clothes that fit properly, consider investing in tailoring. Having your clothes tailored to fit your body perfectly will not only make you look more put-together, but it will also help you feel more confident and comfortable.
By experimenting with trends, accessorizing, paying attention to fit, layering, and investing in tailoring, you can take your look from basic to chic in no time!

SET GOALS AND CRUSH THEM - FIT & SLIM

Staying fit and healthy is a top priority for many people, but it can be challenging to maintain a healthy lifestyle. One of the keys to success is setting achievable goals for yourself and working towards them consistently. In this article, we'll discuss the importance of setting goals and provide tips for crushing them to help you achieve your fitness and weight loss goals.

Why Set Goals?

Setting goals provides a clear direction for your fitness journey and helps you stay motivated. When you have a specific objective in mind, it's easier to make informed decisions about your diet and exercise routine. Additionally, having goals helps you track your progress and stay on track even when you encounter setbacks.

Tips for Setting Effective Goals

Make them Specific: Instead of saying "I want to lose weight," be specific about the amount of weight you want to lose and by when. For example, "I want to lose 10 pounds by the end of next month."

Make them Measurable: Make sure your goals can be tracked and measured. For example, "I want to run a 5K in under 30 minutes."

Make them Achievable: Your goals should be challenging, but also achievable. It's important to avoid setting unrealistic goals that are unlikely to be met, as this can lead to frustration and a lack of motivation.

Make them Relevant: Make sure your goals align with your overall fitness and health goals. For example, if you're trying to lose weight, setting a goal to run a marathon may not be relevant.

Make them Time-bound: Set a deadline for achieving your goals. This helps you stay on track and provides a sense of urgency.

Crushing Your Goals

Now that you have set your goals, it's time to start working towards them. Here are some tips for crushing your goals and achieving success:

Create a Plan: Having a plan in place will help you stay organized and on track. Write down your goals and the steps you need to take to achieve them.

Stay Consistent: Consistency is key when it comes to achieving your goals. Make sure to stick to your plan and avoid making excuses for skipping workouts or eating unhealthy foods.

Track Your Progress: Keeping track of your progress is a great way to stay motivated and see how far you've come. Consider using a fitness app or tracking your progress in a journal.

Stay Positive: It's important to stay positive and focus on the progress you've made, rather than dwelling on setbacks. Celebrate your accomplishments and use them as motivation to keep going.

Surround Yourself with Support: Surrounding yourself with people who support your goals can provide motivation and help you stay on track. Consider joining a fitness group or finding a workout buddy to help keep you accountable.

In conclusion, setting goals is a crucial step in achieving your fitness and weight loss goals. By making your goals specific, measurable, achievable, relevant, and time-bound, you'll have a clear roadmap to success. Stay consistent, track your progress, stay positive, and surround yourself with support to help you crush your goals and achieve your desired outcome.

4 WEEKS FULL BODY WORKOUT CHALLENGE

Week 1 — Focus on your form

Sunday	Lower Body
Monday	Upper Body
Tuesday	Cross Training
Wednesday	Total Body
Thursday	Abs
Friday	Cross Training
Saturday	Rest Time

Week 2 — Go for more reps

Sunday	Lower Body
Monday	Upper Body
Tuesday	Cross Training
Wednesday	Total Body
Thursday	Abs
Friday	Cross Training
Saturday	Rest Time

Week 3 — Try a new cross-training workout

Sunday	Lower Body
Monday	Upper Body
Tuesday	Cross Training
Wednesday	Total Body
Thursday	Abs
Friday	Cross Training
Saturday	Rest Time

Week 4 — Complete and Extra Round

Sunday	Lower Body
Monday	Upper Body
Tuesday	Cross Training
Wednesday	Total Body
Thursday	Abs
Friday	Cross Training
Saturday	Rest Time

Pump it up

BEAUTY WITHOUT HARM!

Go Natural with These Top 7 Healthy Natural Remedies

In today's fast-paced world, it can be tempting to reach for quick and easy solutions to enhance our beauty. However, many of these solutions can contain harmful chemicals and ingredients that can have a negative impact on our health. That's why there's been a growing trend towards a more natural and holistic approach to beauty. In this article, we'll be exploring 5 healthy natural remedies that you can try at home to achieve radiant beauty without harming your health.

Honey and Lemon Face Mask:
This simple and effective face mask is a great way to brighten and clarify your skin. To make the mask, simply mix 1 tablespoon of honey with the juice of half a lemon. Apply the mixture to your face and leave on for 10-15 minutes before rinsing off with warm water. The honey in the mask will hydrate and nourish your skin, while the lemon juice will help to brighten and clarify.

Oatmeal and Yogurt Exfoliating Scrub:
Exfoliating your skin is important for removing dead skin cells and leaving your skin looking and feeling smooth. To make this natural scrub, mix 1/4 cup of oatmeal with 1/4 cup of yogurt to create a paste. Gently massage the mixture onto your face in a circular motion, focusing on areas with dead skin cells. Rinse off with warm water and follow with your usual skincare routine.

Cucumber and Mint Face Mist:
This refreshing face mist is perfect for a quick pick-me-up throughout the day. To make the mist, blend 1 cucumber and a handful of mint leaves together in a blender until smooth. Strain the mixture into a spray bottle and refrigerate. Spritz the mist onto your face to refresh and hydrate your skin.

Avocado and Honey Hair Mask:
Nourishing your hair is just as important as taking care of your skin. To make this hair mask, mash 1 ripe avocado and mix with 1 tablespoon of honey. Apply the mixture to your hair and scalp, making sure to cover all areas. Leave on for 30 minutes before rinsing off with warm water. The avocado in the mask will hydrate and nourish your hair, while the honey will help to make it soft and shiny.

Green Tea and Witch Hazel Toner:
This toner is perfect for balancing your skin's pH, reducing inflammation, and tightening pores. To make the toner, brew 2 green tea bags and let cool. Mix with 2 tablespoons of witch hazel and transfer to a spray bottle. Spritz the toner onto your face after cleansing and before moisturizing.

Prickly Pear Seed Oil Moisturizer: Prickly pear seed oil is rich in antioxidants, essential fatty acids, and vitamin E, making it a great ingredient for skincare. To make this moisturizer, mix 1 tablespoon of prickly pear seed oil with 1 tablespoon of coconut oil and 1 drop of lavender essential oil. Apply a small amount to your face and body each morning and night after cleansing. The prickly pear seed oil in the moisturizer will help to hydrate and nourish your skin, while the coconut oil and lavender essential oil will help to lock in moisture and soothe any irritation.

Black Seed Oil Face Serum:
Black seed oil is rich in antioxidants and anti-inflammatory properties, making it an excellent ingredient for skincare. To make this face serum, mix 1 tablespoon of black seed oil with 1 tablespoon of jojoba oil and 1 drop of vitamin E oil. Apply a small amount to your face each night after cleansing, focusing on areas with fine lines and wrinkles. The black seed oil in the serum will help to hydrate and nourish your skin, while the jojoba oil and vitamin E oil will help to lock in moisture and improve skin elasticity.

You can easily purchase a bottle of high-quality black seed oil on the website www.westendorganix.com.

This recipe is easy to make and use, and it's a great way to incorporate black seed oil into your skincare routine. Give it a try and see how it works for you!

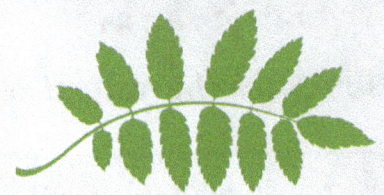

WEST END ORGANIX

Ageless Beauty, Organic Health

BLACK SEED OIL

HEALTHY IMMUNE SYSTEM
INFLAMMATORY RESPONSE

www.westendorganix.com

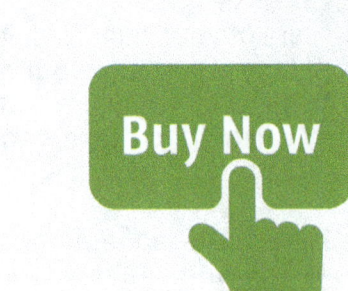

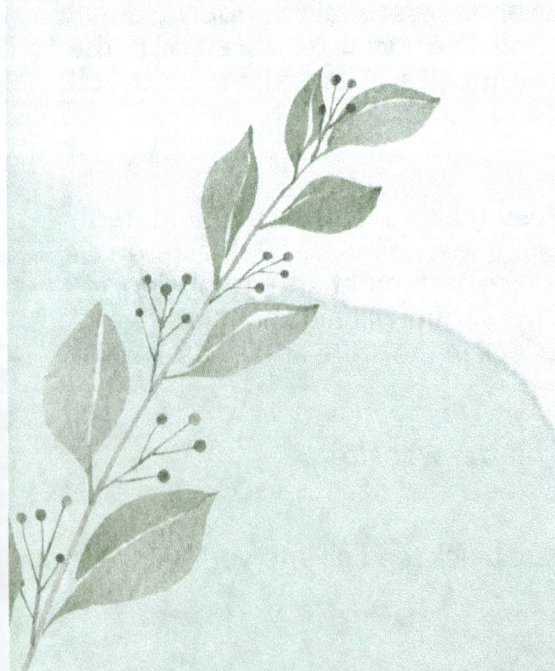

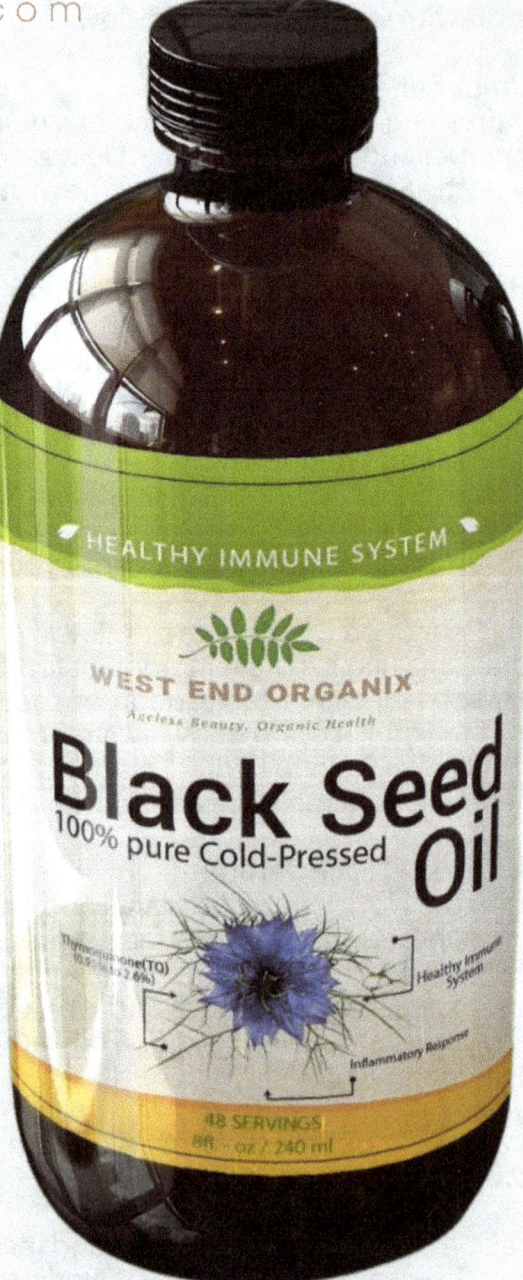

TOP EMPOWERING WOMEN SONGS

A Must-Add Playlist for International Women's Month

Music has the power to inspire and uplift, and there are countless songs that celebrate the strength and resilience of women. In this article, we'll explore the impact of women empowering songs and highlight some of the best tracks that inspire women to embrace their power and confidence.

WHY WOMEN EMPOWERING SONGS ARE IMPORTANT

Women empowering songs play a vital role in promoting gender equality and encouraging women to believe in themselves. These songs celebrate the achievements of women and inspire listeners to break through social and cultural barriers. They also serve as a powerful tool to promote self-esteem and confidence, and remind women of their worth and value.

"I Am Woman" by Helen Reddy - This iconic song, released in 1972, is a feminist anthem that celebrates the strength and courage of women. The lyrics encourage women to stand up for their rights and believe in themselves.

"Survivor" by Destiny's Child - This empowering track, released in 2001, celebrates the resilience of women and encourages listeners to rise above adversity. The lyrics remind women that they are survivors and have the strength to overcome any challenge.

"Roar" by Katy Perry - This upbeat and energetic song, released in 2013, encourages women to embrace their strength and individuality. The lyrics celebrate women who are unafraid to be themselves and stand up for what they believe in.

"Run the World (Girls)" by Beyoncé - This empowering song, released in 2011, celebrates the power and strength of women. The lyrics encourage women to take charge and make their mark on the world.

"Girl on Fire" by Alicia Keys - This uplifting track, released in 2012, celebrates the strength and resilience of women. The lyrics encourage women to break free from their fears and embrace their inner power.

"Gonna Be Alright" by Aneessa" - This uplifting track encourages women to stay strong and have faith in the future, despite any challenges they may face. The lyrics are a powerful reminder that everything will be okay in the end, and that women have the strength and resilience to overcome any obstacle. With its upbeat rhythm and inspiring message, "Gonna Be Alright" is a great addition to any playlist of women empowering songs.

"Fight Song" by Rachel Platten - This empowering track was released in 2015 and has since become an anthem for women everywhere. The lyrics encourage listeners to never give up and to keep fighting for their dreams, no matter what challenges they may face. With its upbeat melody and inspiring message, "Fight Song" is a great addition to any playlist of women empowering songs.

"This Is What You Came For" by Calvin Harris featuring Rihanna- This upbeat EDM track, released in 2016, celebrates the power and confidence of women. The lyrics encourage women to let loose and have fun, and to not hold back or be afraid to be themselves. With its high-energy beat and empowering message, "This Is What You Came For" is a great addition to any playlist of women empowering EDM tracks.

Whether you're looking for an anthem to motivate you to take on the world or a song that celebrates the power of women, these women empowering songs are a must-add to your playlist for International Women's Month.

Listen to the top empowering songs for women on KPIU Radio - the official radio of Pump it Up Magazine! Tune in every day throughout March from 12pm PST to 2pm PST. Visit WWW.KPIURADIO.COM to tune in now!

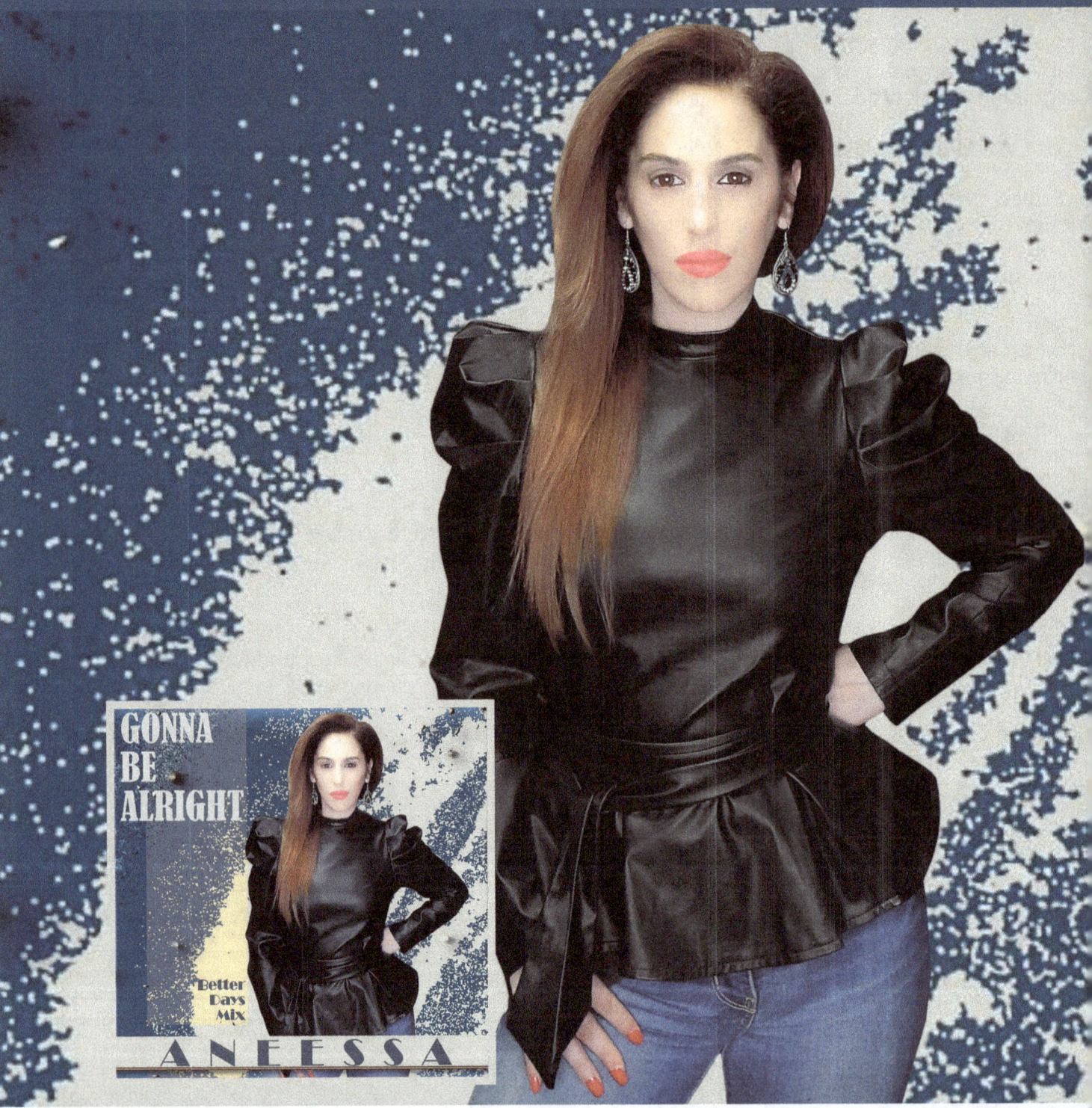

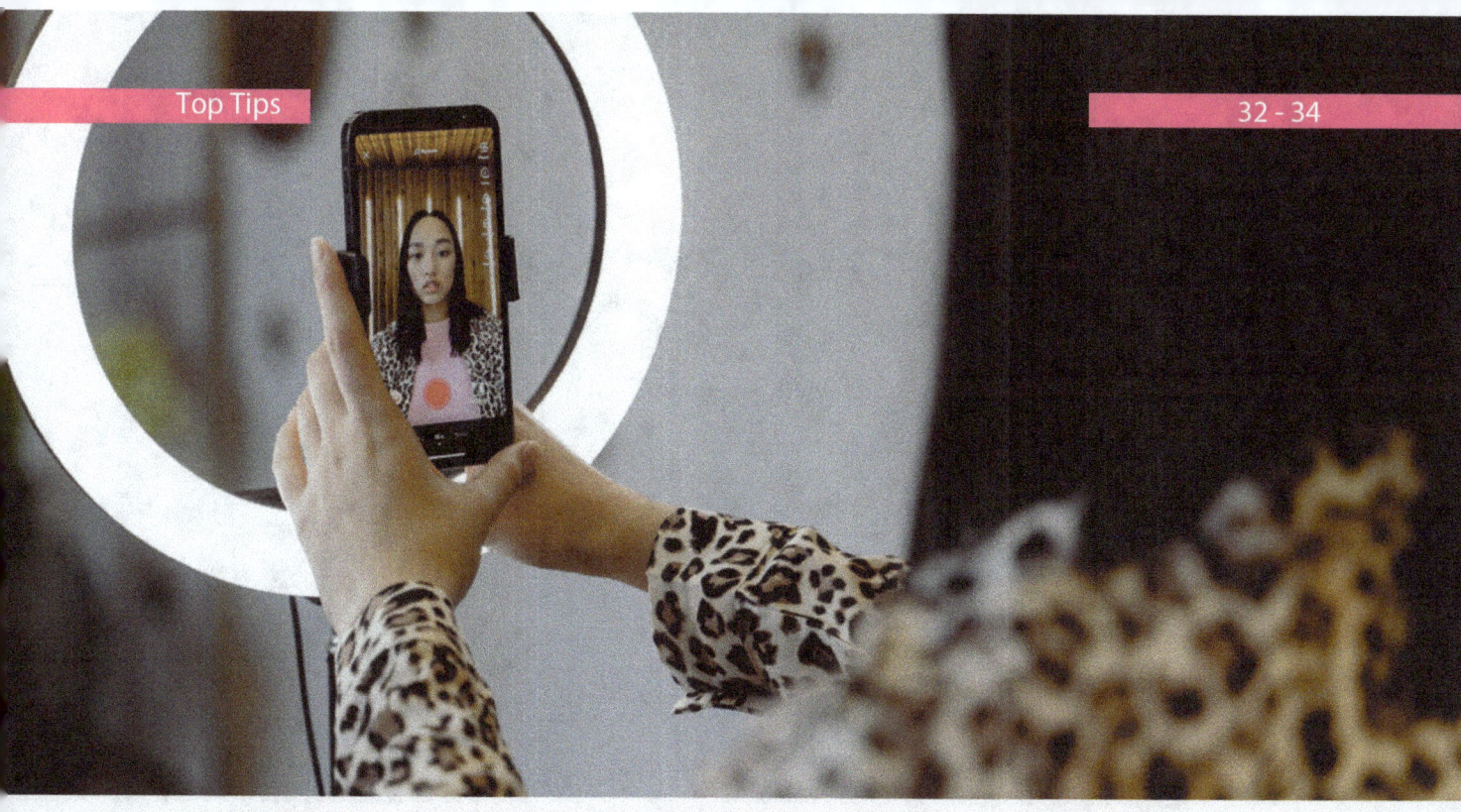

SIMPLE STEPS TO GROW YOUR FOLLOWING
TikTok Tips

TikTok has quickly become one of the most popular social media platforms with millions of users worldwide. If you are looking to grow your following on TikTok, here are some simple steps to help you get started:

Create a niche: TikTok is all about creativity and having a specific niche can help you stand out from the crowd. Choose a topic that you are passionate about and create content that is unique and engaging.

Utilize hashtags: Hashtags are a powerful tool for getting your content discovered on TikTok. Make sure to include relevant hashtags in your posts and participate in trending challenges to reach a larger audience.

Be consistent: Consistency is key when it comes to growing your following on TikTok. Make sure to post regularly and stick to a posting schedule to keep your audience engaged.

Engage with your audience: TikTok is a social platform, which means that engagement is crucial. Respond to comments, participate in challenges and interact with other users to build a strong community around your content.

Make use of TikTok's editing tools: TikTok offers a wide range of editing tools and effects that can help you create eye-catching content. Experiment with different tools and find the ones that work best for you.

Collaborate with other users: Collaborating with other TikTok users can help you reach new audiences and grow your following. Look for users who have a similar niche to yours and reach out to them to collaborate on a project.

Utilize influencer marketing: Influencer marketing can help you reach a larger audience and grow your following on TikTok. Partner with influencers who have a similar niche to yours and work together to create content that will reach a larger audience.

By following these simple steps, you can start to grow your following on TikTok and become a successful creator on the platform.

Good luck!

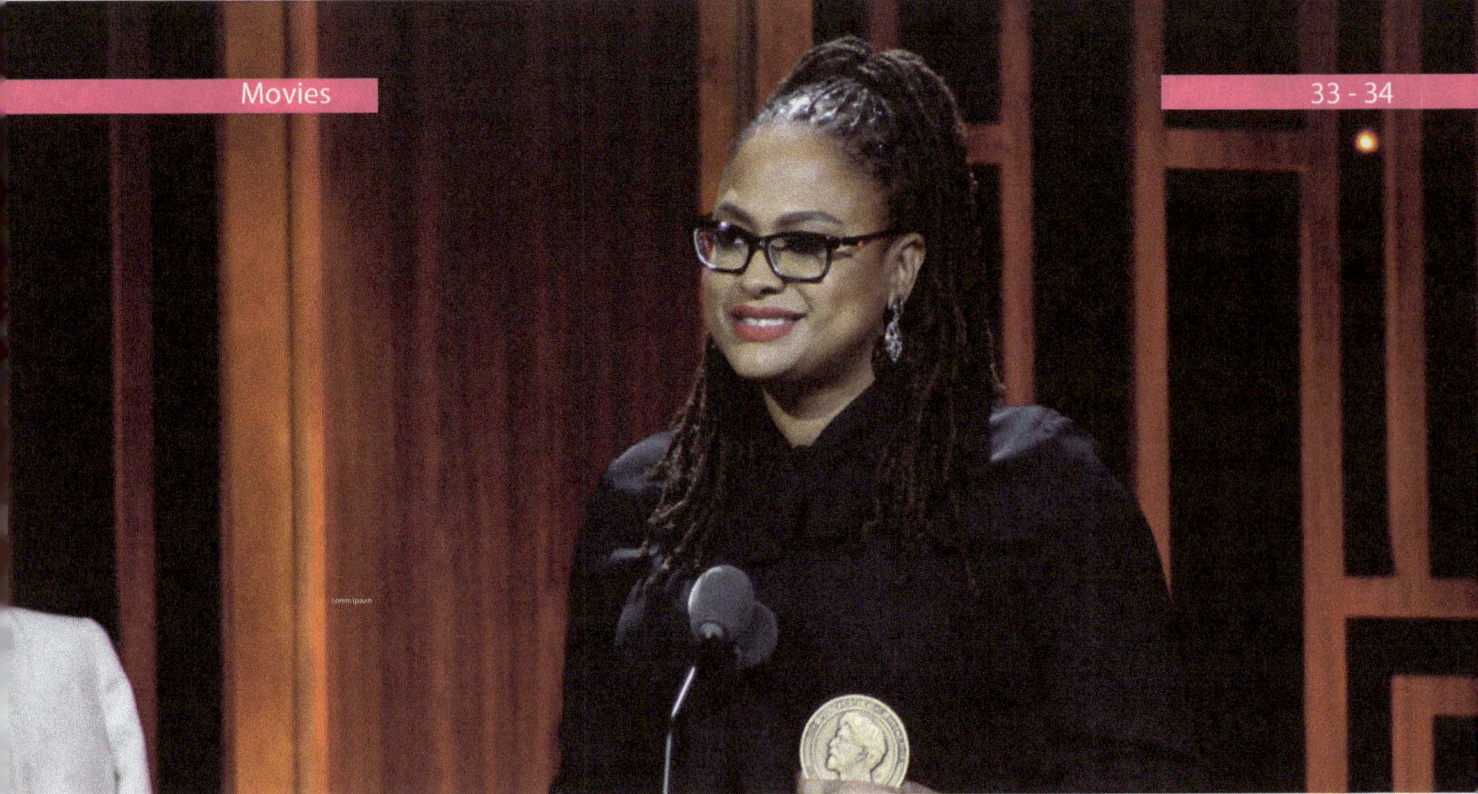

Photo by Stephanie Moreno/Grady College of Journalism and Mass Communications for Peabody Awards/University of Georgia

FEMALE FILMMAKERS MAKING WAVES
Celebrating Women's Contributions to Film on International Women's Day

International Women's Day is a time to celebrate and acknowledge the contributions of women around the world. In the film industry, women have made significant strides in recent years, breaking down barriers and creating compelling stories that captivate audiences. Despite facing ongoing challenges and discrimination, female filmmakers are making waves and changing the landscape of the industry.

One of the most notable female filmmakers of our time is Ava DuVernay, who has made a name for herself with films like "Selma," "13th," and "A Wrinkle in Time." DuVernay is known for her powerful storytelling and her commitment to diversity and representation in her films. She is a trailblazer for women of color in the film industry, and her work has helped to open doors for other female filmmakers.

Another female filmmaker making a big impact is Greta Gerwig, whose films "Lady Bird" and "Little Women" have received widespread critical acclaim. Gerwig's films are known for their strong female characters and their focus on women's experiences and relationships. She has been praised for her writing and her ability to bring a fresh perspective to classic stories.

In recent years, female filmmakers from around the world have been making waves with their unique perspectives and innovative storytelling. From the Middle East, we have directors like Annemarie Jacir, who has explored themes of identity, displacement, and resistance in films like "When I Saw You" and "Wajib." From Africa, we have filmmakers like Wanuri Kahiu, who has pushed boundaries with films like "Rafiki," which was banned in her home country of Kenya for its depiction of a same-sex relationship.

Despite these advances, female filmmakers still face significant challenges in the industry. Women are underrepresented both behind and in front of the camera, and they often receive less funding and support than their male counterparts. However, as more female filmmakers continue to make their mark and tell their stories, the film industry is becoming more diverse and inclusive.

In conclusion, on this International Women's Day, we celebrate the female filmmakers who are making waves and changing the landscape of the film industry. Their contributions to the world of cinema are inspiring, and their work is helping to break down barriers and create a more diverse and inclusive industry. We look forward to seeing what these talented women will achieve in the future.

Do you know of any other female filmmakers who are making a big impact? Share their names and their work on social media and don't forget to tag us too! @pumpitupmagazine

www.ingramcontent.com/pod-product-compliance
Lightning Source LLC
Chambersburg PA
CBHW080901010526
44118CB00015B/2233